GROUP WORK WITH ELDERS

50 Therapeutic Exercises for Reminiscence, Validation, and Remotivation

ANN L. LINK

Professional Resource Press
Sarasota, Florida

Published by Professional Resource Press
(An Imprint of Professional Resource Exchange, Inc.)
Post Office Box 15560
Sarasota, FL 34277-1560

This book was produced in the USA using a patented European binding technology called Otabind. We chose this unique binding because it allows pages to lie flat for photocopying, is stronger than standard bindings for this purpose, and has numerous advantages over spiral binding (e.g., less chance of damage in shipping, no unsightly spiral marks on photocopies, and a spine you can read when the book is on your bookshelf).

The copy editor for this book was Patricia Rockwood, the managing editor was Debbie Fink, the production coordinator was Laurie Girsch, and the cover was created by Carol Tornatore.

Library of Congress Cataloging-in-Publication Data

Link, Ann L., date.
    Group work with elders : 50 therapeutic exercises for
reminiscence, validation, and remotivation / Ann L. Link.
        p.   cm.
    Includes bibliographical references.
    ISBN 1-56887-030-2 (alk. paper)
    1. Group psychotherapy for the aged. 2. Occupational therapy for
the aged. I. Title.
RC451.4.A5L555   1997
618.97' 689152--dc21
                         97-11591
                         CIP

Let's Talk

I roam a landscape of the past,
I wander hallways looking for a friend.
I turn a corner, try a door,
I whisper secrets as I pace the floor.
I long for a familiar smile,
I hide my loneliness behind a yawn.
Come talk with me a little while,
Let's share some tales
Before the day is gone.

Ann Link

DEDICATION

With love and appreciation to my

        parents, family, supportive friends,

               and elder group members

TABLE OF CONTENTS

INTRODUCTION

PURPOSE OF THE BOOK

Group Work with Elders is designed to aid therapists and trained group facilitators who conduct discussion groups for geriatric clients. Exercises in the book combine important geriatric therapy techniques of Reminiscence, Validation, and Remotivation to energize group discussion and foster renewal of hope.

Group participation is a therapeutic tool which is widely supported by experts in the field of geriatrics (Burnside & Schmidt, 1994). Reforms in care for the elderly in skilled nursing facilities have encouraged minimally restrictive forms of treatment (OBRA, 1987). Whenever possible, emotional issues and problem behaviors are treated with methods other than chemical or physical restraints. The majority of reports on group programs for the elderly extol the positive effects of group participation (Toseland, 1990).

BENEFITS OF GROUP

Curative elements of group work described by Yalom (1985) apply to elder populations. The benefit of catharsis, universality, guidance, instillation of hope, group cohesiveness, and interpersonal learning are especially valuable to older group members.

Structured exercises and instructions for group leaders in this book focus on issues pertinent to the aging process, such as coping with loss and decline in independence. Elders who suffer from depression and anxiety may also benefit from a group. In many cases, group participation helps to reduce isolation and lack of relatedness. The exercises are designed to increase feelings of belonging and community. Some group members who have reduced sense of identity and experience confusion may strengthen their reality focus and coping skills through group participation.

WHY A BOOK OF EXERCISES
ESPECIALLY FOR ELDERS?

Although generally seen as beneficial, therapeutic groups for the elderly pose unique difficulties and challenges for the group leader. Members within a group often display varying degrees of cognitive functioning. Some members may suffer from thought disorders or have memory deficits or other limitations to communication or understanding. In addition, older clients sometimes feel threatened by a group discussion format and may resist participating. The exercises presented in this book are designed to ameliorate some of these difficulties. Each exercise has been utilized in geriatric group sessions to monitor for effectiveness and therapeutic value.

Exercises are designed to meet varying needs of group members who function at different cognitive levels. In a heterogeneous group of individuals with various limitations in communication, it is not necessary for each participant to complete every part of an exercise to benefit from the group experience. The elements of the exercises are specifically designed so that each individual in a diversified group may derive some benefit from each exercise. Most exercises are multilevel, including a concrete focus as well as a more abstract concept for group members who appreciate greater complexity. Both pictures and words are featured to stimulate right- and left-brain functions. The use of color and drawing is often suggested to enhance expression. Many exercises include a long-term memory element as well as a here-and-now focus. Memory cues are provided by visual representations and open-ended wording. Large print facilitates easier reading. The use of worksheets helps members with hearing difficulties to follow the exercises. Care has been taken in designing the exercises to maximize participation in a nonthreatening format.

Therapy techniques particularly helpful for elders are emphasized in the instructions for group leaders. Opportunities to validate feelings are presented in each exercise. Cues for reminiscence are frequently employed. A gradual shift to present-day focus within the exercises promotes remotivation and instillation of hope.

SPECIFIC THERAPEUTIC
USES OF THE EXERCISES

VENTILATION AND VALIDATION OF FEELINGS

Group participation helps to validate and affirm the feelings and experiences of older adults (Toseland, 1990). Interacting with peers who express similar concerns and emotional reactions encourages group members in their efforts to cope with adverse life experiences. Feeling heard, understood, and accepted are major building blocks to self-esteem in the elderly. Relating to the emotional tone of communication is often more important than focusing on content (Feil, 1992).

REMINISCENCE

Exercises in this book frequently trigger reminiscence, which is a valuable tool in helping the elderly client review life events to gain perspective, derive meaning, and work toward resolution (Burnside & Schmidt, 1994). Erickson (1982) describes the task of later life as developing integrity and wisdom versus despair. Members share past accomplishments, explore disappointments, and arrive at new viewpoints. Reminiscence in a group of peers helps to build group cohesion and feelings of belonging.

REMOTIVATION AND INSTILLATION OF HOPE

The elderly person in a residential setting often has difficulty investing interest in his or her present environment, which leads to feelings of isolation and hopelessness. During supportive group interaction, members become better acquainted with each other and increase their awareness of possible interests and activities available in their living situation. Positive group interaction can increase motivation and a sense of hope (Robinson, n.d.). Structured exercises are designed to stimulate interaction and broaden awareness.

INTERPERSONAL LEARNING

Coping with stress is a never-ending life task. Reviewing past coping skills encourages members in their efforts to deal with frustration and adapt to change (Toseland, 1990). Listening to others in a group discussion describe coping skills and survival techniques promotes interpersonal learning. Opportunities are presented in the exercises to practice coping behavior in a supportive atmosphere.

GROUP COHESION AND RELATEDNESS

Loss of loved ones and weakening of social ties often lead to feelings of worthlessness and isolation for the elderly. Making new connections with people is difficult; however, feelings of relatedness and belonging enhance self-esteem and increase motivation for living. The exercises presented in this book are designed to foster group cohesion and interaction in a nonthreatening, therapeutic format.

SUGGESTIONS AND PRECAUTIONS
FOR GROUP LEADERS

INTRODUCTION TO THE GROUP

Many elders are not open to the idea of a mental health therapy group, feeling that there is a stigma attached to participation. Members often prefer to call the group a "class" or simply a "discussion group." The purpose of the group might be explained as an opportunity to share ideas and learn from each other's experiences.

SELECTION OF MEMBERS

Although a structured group process can sustain varying levels of cognitive functioning and is beneficial for many elders, it is not appropriate for everyone. Group participation may be counterproductive for highly disruptive individuals, persons who cannot allow others to have their turn at speaking, or members who wander off while the group is in session.

GROUP SETTING

Seating around a square or round table where members can see each other is recommended. A private or semiprivate atmosphere encourages disclosure. Some group leaders include a snack or beverage at the end of the session to encourage relatedness and a sense of belonging.

GROUP FORMAT

Structured group formats are often effective for geriatric populations because they generate interaction, provide focus, stimulate reminiscence, and promote inclusion. Flexibility should allow for unstructured discussion as well. Some leaders alternate structured groups with unstructured groups. Other leaders allow time at the beginning of each group session to deal with immediate concerns of group members, such as illness, situational events, natural disasters, and so forth. It is important to stay in touch with the needs of group members to insure that the group experience is relevant and valuable.

CONFIDENTIALITY

Members are encouraged to respect each other's privacy and refrain from revealing information learned within the group to persons outside the group.

GROUP LEADER'S ROLE

Inclusion is very important in working with the elderly in groups (Burnside & Schmidt, 1994). Each member should be welcomed at every session, and members' names should be used profusely throughout the sessions. The leader should be instrumental in preventing any individual from dominating the group. Each member should have an opportunity to contribute to the discussion. Group members should be encouraged, but not pressured, to participate in the exercises. Members need to feel in control of how much or how little they divulge.

Each contribution should be acknowledged. Modeling a supportive, accepting attitude while maintaining appropriate boundaries and structure is a key element to successful group leadership and may help members to generalize these attitudes outside of the group.

MEMBERS WITH IMPAIRMENTS

Many groups for the elderly will include members who have some degree of impairment which impedes communication. The goal of the group leader is to enhance individual participation to maximize each member's potential for interaction. It may not be realistic that each member relate to every aspect of an exercise. A more realistic goal is to use techniques in leading the group that maximize each individual's potential for interaction. Some members will benefit from the entire scope of an exercise, while other members may relate only to a portion of the exercise, such as reminiscence connected to the illustration. It is imperative that the leader model an accepting attitude toward individual differences. This is accomplished by focusing on the member's contribution rather than directing attention to some part of the exercise the member has not been able to complete. For example, if a group member declines to complete most of an exercise, but colors some part of the illustration, the leader may encourage interaction by saying something like: "Mary, I notice that you have colored the roof of the well red. I'm wondering if this has some special meaning for you?" Mary, in turn, may respond with reminiscence of a red-roofed well in her past. The feeling tone of colors and drawings can be commented on in a supportive manner, making sure to always check out the validity of impressions with the group member. It is important to emphasize the importance of expression of feelings rather than artistic talent (Oster & Gould, 1987). Drawing and color enhance communication, but each exercise can also be used effectively with verbal or written participation.

A main function of a therapeutic group is to foster meaningful interaction and a sense of belonging. Exercise sheets are to be used as a guide and stimulus for participation, not as mandatory assignments. Members may fill out as much or as little of an exercise sheet as they desire. Whether or not they read or write, each member is given an exercise sheet as a symbol of inclusion. Words are provided in the exercises for those who like to read and write. In some cases, members respond more fully by writing than by talking. It is important to describe pictures and read sentences aloud to include members who do not see well or cannot read or write. These individuals are included in the discussion as members are encouraged to share their ideas verbally.

Persons who are hard of hearing often appreciate visual and written guidelines included in the exercise sheets. These members may also be seated near the leader to facilitate hearing. It is always important for the leader to speak clearly and distinctly, repeating questions and directions as needed.

CONFUSED OR DELUSIONAL MEMBERS

Severely disturbed individuals who cannot focus and who interrupt others continually are not appropriate for inclusion in a group. Members who are able to focus to some extent and are moderately confused or delusional can benefit from a group if the leader provides appropriate structure and support. Most exercises feature a concrete, familiar topic to help strengthen a reality focus; thus, if a confused group member strays from the topic, bringing up unrelated or delusional ideas, the leader may gently redirect the discussion back to the topic. For example, the leader might respond, "Bob, you have described ideas about spacemen. Today our topic is food. Can you name some foods you like?"

If the delusional response refers to the topic, the leader can show understanding for the feeling tone of the response without directly confirming or disputing the content of the remark. For example, Alice may assert that her mother poisoned the family's bread when she baked. The leader might respond, "Alice, it sounds like you felt distrustful of eating bread your mother baked." The leader may also redirect toward a positive focus by asking questions, such as, "Was there any bread you felt comfortable eating?" or "When did you enjoy eating bread?" Directly disputing a delusional response may cause a member to feel misunderstood and defensive. Acknowledging the emotion behind a delusional statement provides support and encourages communication (Feil, 1992).

MEMORY PROBLEMS

It is important that the group leader deal with participants' memory problems in a supportive manner to lessen feelings of inadequacy. Several techniques are helpful in maintaining participation when a group member cannot recall something asked for in an exercise. The leader can ask for voluntary responses by asking, "Who would like to share a memory they have about baking bread?" Members who do not respond to this question may be asked related questions that do not require as much memory, such as, "Mary, do you like bread with your meals?" Asking questions in a multiple-choice format helps to trigger memories; for example, the leader may encourage a response by asking, "Bob, which do you like better, home-baked bread or store-bought bread?" (Feil, 1992).

Another technique that encourages responses is to involve the group. For example, if a member is asked to name a romantic person and responds, "I don't know" or "I don't remember," the leader may ask the group for help by saying, "Who can suggest people Alice may have found romantic?" Suggestions might include Alice's husband, Clark Gable, and so on. The leader then thanks the group for their suggestions and asks Alice if any of the suggestions match her idea of a romantic person. This is a variation on the multiple-choice format that often elicits a response. It is helpful to remember that the most important function of any exercise is to encourage expression and a feeling of belonging.

CONCLUSION

Leading groups for geriatrics is greatly facilitated by use of *Group Work with Elders.* Complex psychological tasks of aging deserve the special emphasis featured in this book. Coming to terms with the meaning of life in its final stages can be lonely and overwhelming. Meeting with others to share feelings, experiences, and ideas for coping reduces isolation and despair. Facilitating groups for geriatrics is a rewarding challenge when the group process is used to inspire elders in their psychological struggle to attain integrity and dignity.

REFERENCES

Burnside, I., & Schmidt, M. (1994). *Working with Older Adults, Group Process and Techniques.* Boston: Jones and Bartlett.

Erickson, E. (1982). *The Life Cycle Completed.* New York: W. W. Norton and Company.

Feil, N. (1992). *V/F Validation: The Feil Method (rev. ed.).* Cleveland, OH: Edward Feil Productions, 4614 Prospect Avenue, Cleveland, OH 44103.

Omnibus Budget Reconciliation Act of 1987 (OBRA, 1987). Amendments to Title XIX of the Social Security Act, Sections 1819 & 1919, b.4.

Oster, G., & Gould, P. (1987). *Using Drawings in Assessment and Therapy.* New York: Brunner/Mazel.

Robinson, A. M. (n.d.). *Remotivation Techniques: A Manual for Use in Nursing Homes.* Philadelphia: American Psychiatric Association and Smith, Kline & French Laboratories Remotivation Project.

Toseland, R. (1990). *Group Work with Older Adults.* New York: University Press.

Yalom, I. D. (1985). *The Theory and Practice of Group Psychotherapy (3rd ed.).* New York: Basic Books.

GROUP WORK WITH ELDERS

50 Therapeutic Exercises for Reminiscence, Validation, and Remotivation

Exercise 1

FOODS AND FEELINGS

Purpose:

1. Stimulate positive reminiscence about foods.
2. Explore feelings about current foods eaten.

Materials:

One photocopy of illustration for each group member; pencils, fine-line colored felt pens, or crayons.

Procedure:

A. While handing out materials, the leader asks members to think about home-cooked meals they have enjoyed.
B. Those who wish may draw a favorite dinner cooking on the stove or in the oven. Some members may want to color the illustration.
C. The sentences below the illustration are read aloud. Members are asked to complete the sentences.

Group Discussion:

Members are asked to share memories about stoves similar to the one in the illustration. The leader asks questions, such as whether members recall where the wood or coal was burned in the stove, and how the water was heated.

Members share their illustrations and responses to the questions. If members share frustrations about current diets, the leader asks how other group members cope with similar frustrations. Ideas for coping might include communicating about dietary likes and dislikes, finding out more about the purpose of dietary restrictions, and use of substitutions which are allowed in the members' diet. Members are also encouraged to talk about foods in their current diet that they enjoy to increase positive feelings about mealtimes.

Sharing ideas about a familiar subject in a nonthreatening format helps group members to express feelings, develop trust, and build feelings of community.

Foods and Feelings

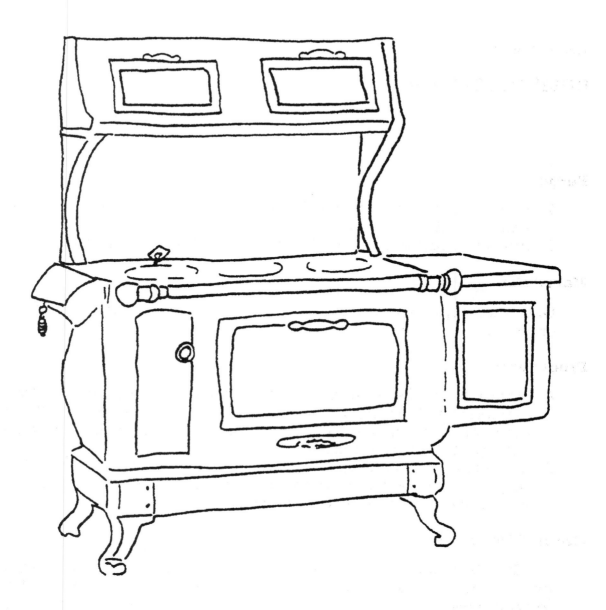

A home-cooked meal I like: _____

_____

Food I like now: _____

If I could change the food I eat now I would: _____

_____

_____

Exercise 2

COMMUNICATION

Purpose:

1. Encourage expression of feelings regarding communication in the past and present.
2. Provide group support for feelings of loneliness or isolation.

Materials:

One photocopy of the illustration for each group member; pencils and crayons.

Procedure:

A. Materials are distributed and the leader asks group members to share memories and associations related to the phones in the illustration. Some members may recall talking on a party line and even remember their party-line phone signal.
B. Members are encouraged to complete the sentences. Some members may wish to color the illustration or draw the face of a person they would like to talk to next to the receiver.

Group Discussion:

Members share their illustrations and ideas about people they would like to contact. Members are asked to tell about losing contact with people in their lives and how they feel about these experiences. The leader asks the group for ideas on ways to maintain contact with others.

This exercise is helpful in stimulating interest in communication and allowing ventilation of feelings regarding loss and isolation.

Variations:

Group members are encouraged to plan one way to communicate with someone they would like to contact. In later meetings, members may wish to share their experiences.

Communication

I would like to talk to: _____

I would talk about: _____

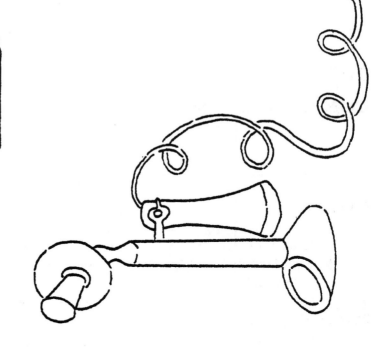

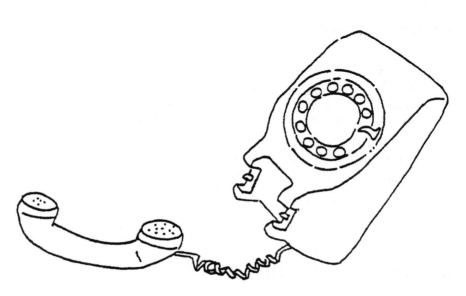

Exercise 3

ROMANTIC MOMENTS

Purpose:

1. Share personal memories and feelings to increase a sense of belonging.
2. Practice reminiscence in a group setting to strengthen identity and self-esteem.

Materials:

One photocopy of the illustration for each group member; crayons and pencils.

Procedure:

A. While materials are being distributed, the leader asks members to think about romantic moments in their lives.
B. The sentence fragments are read aloud and members are asked to fill in the blanks. Members are told they can write about events in their own lives or romantic scenes from a book or movie.
C. Members who wish may draw favorite candies in the box and color the box.

Group Discussion:

Members share their illustrations and sentences. If members share frustrations or feelings of loss about a disappointing romance, the leader and other group members offer support by expressing feelings of understanding and empathy.

This exercise increases group cohesiveness by stimulating reminiscence and promoting expression of feelings. Participants may discover that other group members share their interest in particular movie stars. Sharing common interests helps to build relatedness.

Romantic Moments

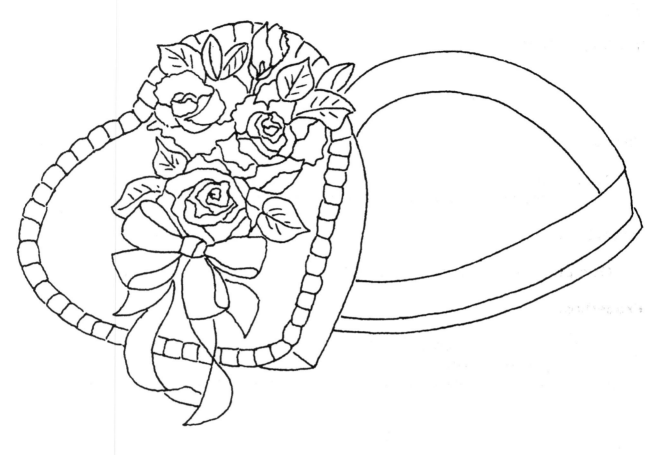

_____ was a very romantic person.

A favorite romantic memory of mine: _____

_____

_____

_____

A romantic movie star: _____

_____

_____

Exercise 4

TRANSPORTATION

Purpose:

1. Encourage expression of feelings about mobility and independence.
2. Promote active listening and awareness of the feelings of others.

Materials:

One photocopy of the illustration for each member; pencils and crayons.

Procedure:

A. Members are asked to think about their favorite car while materials are being passed out.
B. The sentence fragments are read aloud and members are asked to fill in the blanks.
C. Members who wish may draw someone in the car, color the car, or draw a favorite car design of their own.

Group Discussion:

Members share their illustrations and sentences. Members who did not drive are asked how they managed transportation.

Members are encouraged to share memories and feelings about the Model T in the illustration.

Members are asked how transportation is managed where they live. If feelings of frustration about transportation are expressed, the leader and group members may provide group support by validating feelings and offering suggestions for coping.

This exercise is beneficial in stimulating group support and encouraging ventilation of frustrations about declines in independence.

Transportation

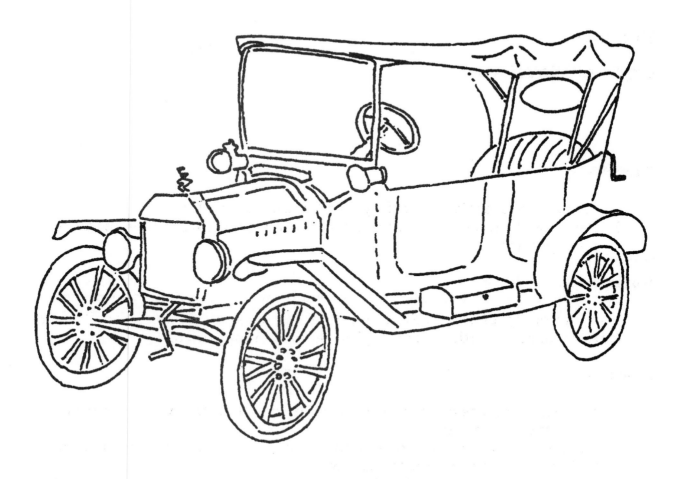

My favorite car: _____

_____

A car I would like to have driven: _____

_____

Exercise 5

GROUP POEM

Purpose:

1. Promote expression of feelings and enhance creativity.
2. Raise self-esteem and group morale by contributing to a collective creative project.

Materials:

One photocopy of Group Poem worksheet for each member; pencils. **Optional:** posterboard, scissors, glue, and old magazines.

Procedure:

A. The leader points out that we are each unique in the way we experience and express feelings.
B. Materials are distributed and the leader explains that the photocopy will be used to create a group poem.
C. Members are instructed to finish the sentences on the worksheet. The leader may help those who have difficulty writing.

Group Discussion:

Members take turns reading and discussing their contributions. Permission is asked of the members to combine their expressions into a poem. Using the group leader's worksheet, the leader arranges the various ideas supplied by the members to complete a poem. Copies are distributed to the members acknowledging their special contributions.

This exercise increases feelings of belonging and promotes good self-esteem. Members are often pleased by how their contributions add to the effectiveness of the poem.

Variation:

The group poem can be displayed on posterboard. Pictures from old magazines can be cut out and glued around a copy of the poem to illustrate the ideas in the poem.

Group Poem

Fall leaves remind me of:

_____

When winter comes, I feel:

_____

When spring comes, I hope for:

_____

My favorite flower:

_____

It's good to think about:

_____

Group Leader's Worksheet for Group Poem

Fall leaves remind me of:

_____

_____

_____

_____

_____

When winter comes, I feel:

_____

_____

_____

_____

_____

When spring comes, I hope for:

_____

_____

_____

_____

_____

My favorite flower:

_____

_____

_____

_____

_____

It's good to think about:

_____

_____

_____

_____

_____

Exercise 6

COPING WITH PAIN

Purpose:

1. Promote healthy mechanisms for coping with pain or disability.
2. Increase understanding of and group support for meeting health challenges.

Materials:

One photocopy of the illustration for each group member; crayons.

Procedure:

A. Materials are distributed and the leader explains that the figures in the illustration represent the front and back of a patient arriving for and leaving a doctor's appointment.
B. Members are asked to think about physical pain they have experienced. Members are instructed to select colors to represent pain or limitation they experience or have experienced and color the corresponding part on the figures in the drawing.

Group Discussion:

Members present their figures and tell about the pain in the areas they have colored. Members are asked what they do to cope with pain or disability. Their answers may give other group members ideas on how to cope.

This exercise promotes empathy and bonding in older populations who are particularly stressed by physical problems. Participants may become more aware of the physical challenges others face and consequently develop greater empathy for others.

Coping With Pain

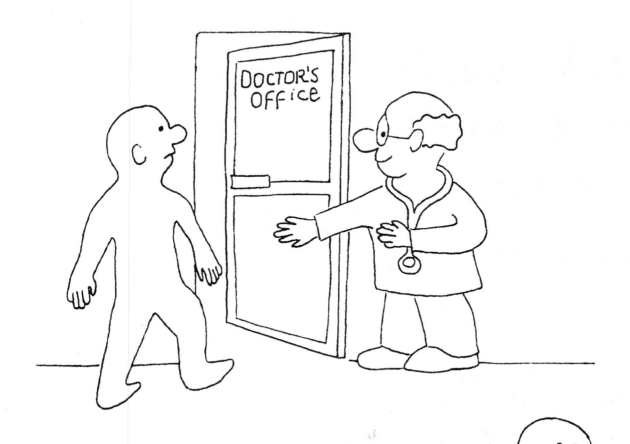

Physical pain that bothers me the most:

_____

_____

I try to cope with pain by: _____

_____

_____

Exercise 7

WISH ON A STAR

Purpose:

1. Explore feelings about past and present wishes.
2. Increase understanding of the needs of others and universality of common concerns.

Materials:

One photocopy of the illustration for each member; pencils and crayons.

Procedure:

A. While materials are being handed out, members are asked to think about things they wished for as a child.
B. The leader or a group member reads the poem. Members are asked to share memories about the poem and about childhood wishes.
C. The leader asks members to list three present-day wishes in the blanks. Members may color the picture if they wish.

Group Discussion:

Members share their illustrations and wishes. The leader asks members if they see a difference between their childhood wishes and their present-day wishes. The leader points out common themes expressed in the wishes, such as desires for independence, security, and companionship.

Sharing about common needs in this exercise helps to build a feeling of community and belonging.

Wish on a Star

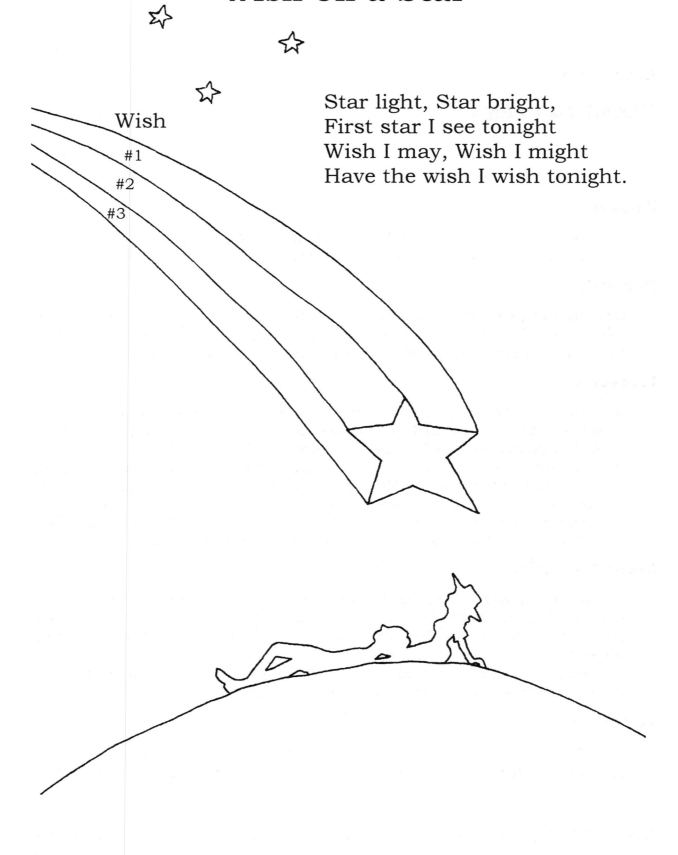

Wish

#1

#2

#3

Star light, Star bright,
First star I see tonight
Wish I may, Wish I might
Have the wish I wish tonight.

Exercise 8

THANK-YOU CARD

Purpose:

    1. Develop appreciation for the contributions of others.
    2. Practice social skill of expressing appreciation.

Materials:

One photocopy of the illustration for each member, folded in half and then folded in half again to form a greeting card; pencils or pens or fine-line colored felt pens. ***Optional:*** small pieces of paper and a hat or box.

Procedure:

    A. While materials are being distributed, the leader explains that the hand-out is a thank-you card. The leader points out that most people like to feel appreciated, but it is easy to forget to thank others.
    B. The members are asked to suggest people in their living environment who might appreciate a thank-you card. Suggestions might include cooks, housekeepers, and gardeners.
    C. Members are asked to color flowers on the empty stems and sign their name inside the card. Some members may want to write a message.

Group Discussion:

    Members show their cards and tell who they would like to give the card to and why they chose that person. Suggestions are given to members who want to give their card to someone, but don't know how to go about it.

    Practicing the social skill of expressing appreciation in a safe environment promotes relatedness and positive interaction.

Variation:

    Members may draw each other's names out of a hat and give their card to a group member. This variation helps to build group cohesion.

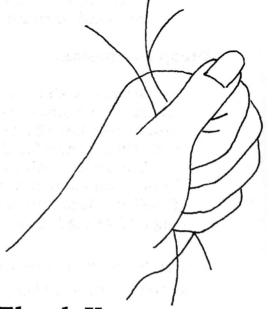

Thank You

Exercise 9

FAMILY BACKGROUNDS

Purpose:

1. Promote greater understanding of self and others by sharing family backgrounds.
2. Increase trust by practicing self-disclosure in a supportive atmosphere.

Materials:

One photocopy of the illustration for each member; pencils or fine-line colored felt pens.

Procedure:

A. Members are given a photocopy of the picture frame and asked to draw their birth family. The leader emphasizes that drawing ability is not important. Members who have difficulty drawing may use circles or stick figures to represent family members.
B. The leader explains that a person's position in the family as oldest, youngest, or middle child often affects the role the person plays in the family. The leader gives examples, such as an older child being put in charge of things, or a youngest child being overprotected. Members are asked to think about the role they played in their family.

Group Discussion:

Members show their family drawings and tell about their position in the family as oldest, youngest, or middle child. Each person is asked how family position affected relationships with parents and siblings. Members are asked if their family position still affects how they interact with people.

The leader points out similarities among the families of group members, such as members who were oldest children, or members from large families. Becoming aware of similarities helps to build a sense of belonging and relatedness.

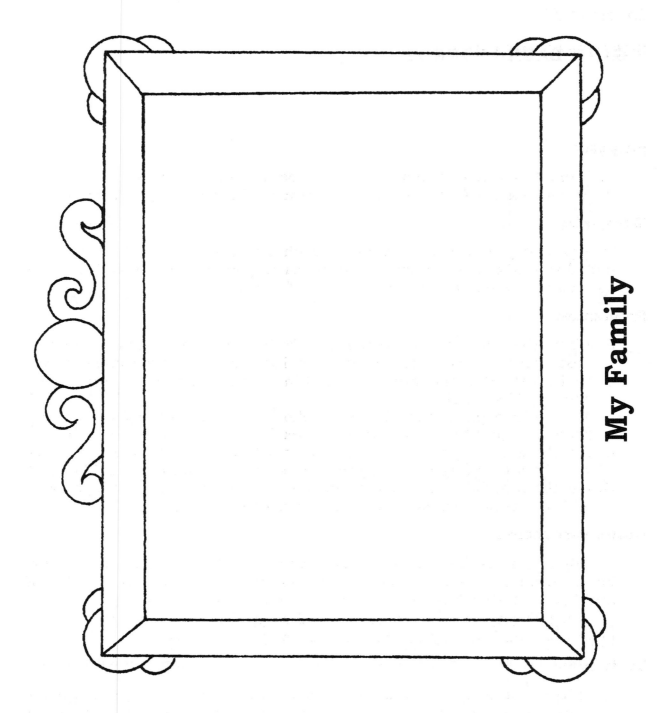

My Family

Exercise 10

WISHING YOU LUCK

Purpose:

    1. Promote group cohesion by sharing personal information.
    2. Encourage consideration and awareness of the feelings of others.

Materials:

One photocopy of the illustration for each member, folded in half and then folded in half again to form a greeting card; pens or pencils and fine-line colored felt pens; hat or box and slips of paper.

Procedure:

    A. While the materials are being distributed, the leader points out that most people have experienced good luck and bad luck sometime in their lives. Members are asked to think about their own experiences of good and bad luck.
    B. The leader explains that the folded photocopy is a card to wish someone good luck, and that members will be exchanging cards with each other.
    C. Members are instructed to color the card, draw something associated with luck in the space above the pot, and sign their name to the card.
    D. Members draw each other's names out of a hat and exchange cards with the person whose name they have drawn.

Group Discussion:

Members display the card they have received and reveal which member gave them the card. Members are asked to share stories about good and bad luck they have experienced in their lives.

Exchanging cards wishing each other good luck encourages feelings of goodwill and belonging which increases group cohesion.

Variation:

If drawing names from a hat is too confusing for some groups, members can pass their card to a member on their right instead of drawing names.

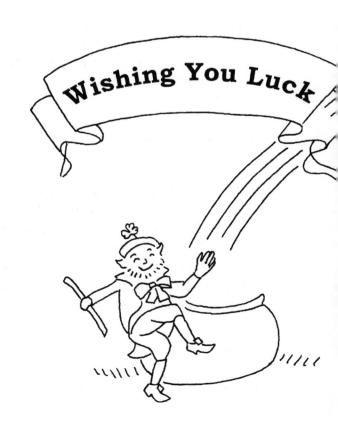
Wishing You Luck

Exercise 11

THE AMERICAN FLAG

Purpose:

1. Increase understanding and tolerance of others.
2. Promote group cohesion by sharing feelings about a common theme.

Materials:

One photocopy of the illustration for each group member; pencils, crayons, or fine-line colored felt pens. ***Optional:*** large piece of dark blue posterboard; scissors and glue.

Procedure:

A. Materials are handed out. The leader explains that, depending on a person's background, living in the United States has different meanings.
B. The statement is read aloud. Members are instructed to write their ideas about what living in the United States means to them.
C. Members are asked to think of things that remind them of the flag and draw those things around the flag. Members are encouraged to color their pictures.

Group Discussion:

Members share their pictures and ideas about living in the United States. The leader asks if anyone has visited or lived in another country and their reactions to other countries. Members are asked if they have served in the armed forces and how they feel about that experience.

This exercise helps group members to become better acquainted and develop better understanding of each other. Discussions about the flag are especially appropriate around July 4th, Veteran's Day, or Flag Day; however, this exercise can be useful any time of year.

Variation:

The colored flag designs and the members' original drawings can be cut out and glued onto dark blue posterboard to form a patriotic poster labeled, "What living in the United States means to me."

The American Flag

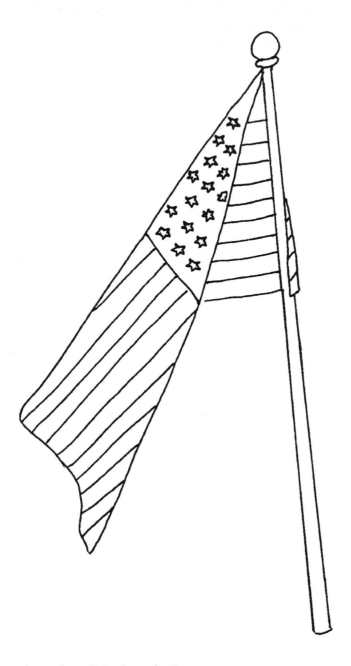

What living in the United States means to me: _____

_____

_____

_____

_____

Exercise 12

THE BEST THING SINCE SLICED BREAD

Purpose:

1. Promote group cohesiveness by sharing feelings about a common subject in a nonthreatening format.
2. Stimulate reminiscence about significant personal history.

Materials:

One photocopy of the illustration for each group member; pencils and crayons.

Procedure:

A. Materials are handed out and the quotation is read aloud. Members are asked if they have heard the saying "The best thing since sliced bread," and what they think the saying means.
B. Members are asked to write down one or more memories involving bread.
C. Members who wish may color the pictures and add drawings of special breads they remember.

Group Discussion:

Members show their pictures and share reminiscences about bread, such as memories of their mother baking bread. Sharing memories about a common, nonthreatening theme helps to build a sense of belonging.

The leader explains that the saying "The best thing since sliced bread" refers to an innovation or invention that is as important as the advent of presliced bread. Members are asked to name something invented since their childhood that they especially appreciate, such as electric dishwashers or television.

This exercise helps to build feelings of belonging, because group members may have experiences in common adjusting to innovations and inventions in their lifetimes.

The Best Thing
Since Sliced Bread

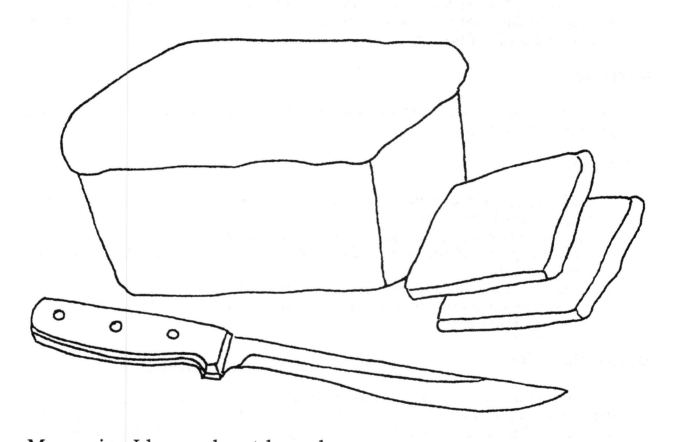

Memories I have about bread: _____

_____

_____

_____

_____

Exercise 13

MY HOME STATE

Purpose:

1. Enhance identity and self-esteem by sharing personal history.
2. Promote interpersonal awareness by increasing knowledge about the backgrounds of others.

Materials:

One photocopy of U.S. map for each group member and one for the leader; pencils and crayons.

Procedure:

A. While materials are being handed out, members are asked to think about their home state.
B. The leader explains that growing-up experiences in different states and different parts of the world affect how people feel about their current living situation.
C. Members are asked to initial and color their home state. If members cannot recall their home state, they can color and initial their present state of residence.

Group Discussion:

One at a time, members share their pictures and information about their home state. Members may reminisce about weather, industries, crops, or seasonal activities of their home state. As each member reveals this information, the group leader fills in a map by writing the member's name on the appropriate state to form a combined map. The combined map is displayed to illustrate which states are represented by various group members.

Members are encouraged to share how they feel about their current state of residence and how they felt about moving from their home state.

Members who have lived in the same state all of their lives can share how they feel about this and whether they would have enjoyed living elsewhere.

This exercise helps to increase awareness of others. The leader can emphasize similarities and differences of members' backgrounds to encourage relatedness.

My Home State

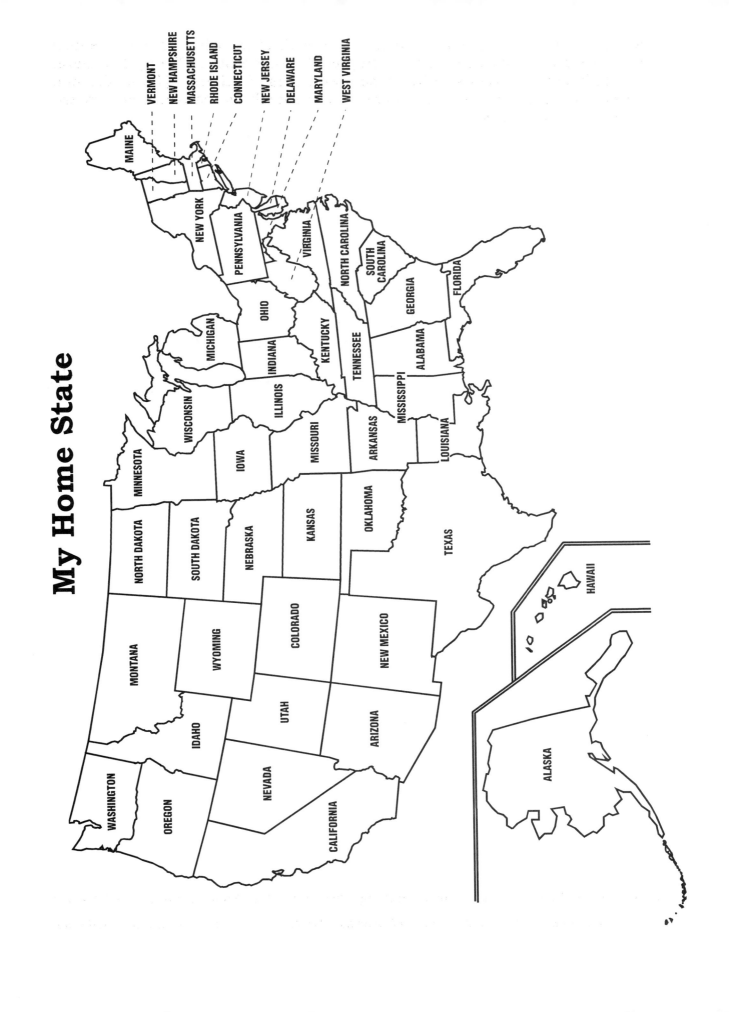

VERMONT
NEW HAMPSHIRE
MASSACHUSETTS
RHODE ISLAND
CONNECTICUT
NEW JERSEY
DELAWARE
MARYLAND
WEST VIRGINIA

MAINE
NEW YORK
PENNSYLVANIA
VIRGINIA
NORTH CAROLINA
SOUTH CAROLINA
FLORIDA
OHIO
KENTUCKY
TENNESSEE
GEORGIA
ALABAMA
MISSISSIPPI
MICHIGAN
INDIANA
ILLINOIS
WISCONSIN
MISSOURI
ARKANSAS
LOUISIANA
IOWA
MINNESOTA
NORTH DAKOTA
SOUTH DAKOTA
NEBRASKA
KANSAS
OKLAHOMA
TEXAS
COLORADO
NEW MEXICO
WYOMING
MONTANA
IDAHO
UTAH
ARIZONA
NEVADA
WASHINGTON
OREGON
CALIFORNIA
HAWAII
ALASKA

Exercise 14

SETTING BOUNDARIES

Purpose:

1. Encourage ventilation of feelings.
2. Provide group support in coping effectively.

Materials:

One photocopy of the illustration for each member; pencils and crayons.

Procedure:

A. Materials are distributed and the sentence fragments are read aloud.
B. Members are asked to think about a time when someone intruded on their space and how they felt about this.
C. Members are instructed to complete the sentences. They may color the picture if they wish.

Group Discussion:

Members read their sentences and share feelings about experiences in the past and present when someone has not respected their personal space or possessions. Members are encouraged to describe their feelings and how they coped with intrusions. The leader helps members define appropriate boundaries and develop positive coping techniques.

Older individuals in a group living situation often feel frustrated by the lack of privacy. Airing feelings in a supportive group setting may help to strengthen coping skills.

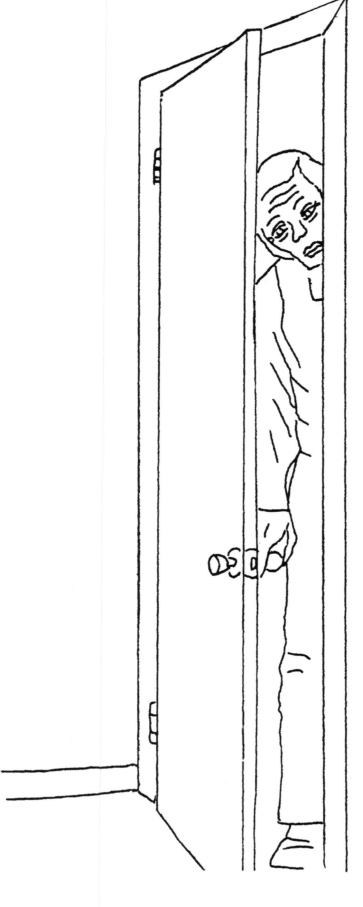

Setting
Boundaries

When someone invades
my space, I feel: _____

_____

_____

_____

_____

The best way to handle
this is to: _____

_____

_____

_____

Exercise 15:

RELAXATION

Purpose:

1. Teach techniques to promote relaxation.
2. Increase relatedness by sharing personal information.

Materials:

One photocopy of the illustration for each member; pencils and crayons.

Procedure:

A. Group leader explains that relaxation promotes stress reduction and positive coping.
B. Members are given copies of the illustration and asked to write down a relaxing place or draw themselves in a scene they find relaxing. Members may color the scene if they prefer.
C. Group members are asked to participate in the following relaxation exercise:

> Clench both hands tightly while I count slowly to 5. 1 . . . 2 . . . 3 . . . 4 . . . 5. Now relax your hands completely. Close your eyes. Take a deep breath. Let the air out slowly. Each time you breathe out, let troubles and worries leave your body. Allow your body to relax completely. Imagine a place that is relaxing for you. Picture the colors and textures. Imagine the small details of this relaxing place. Allow peace and relaxation to permeate your body. Allow yourself to relax more and more. Imagine that you can bring this peaceful feeling with you to any setting by imagining a relaxing scene and reminding yourself to relax . . . relax. Bring this feeling of relaxation with you now back to our group meeting. Slowly open your eyes as I count to 3. 1 . . . 2 . . . 3.

Group Discussion:

Members share their experiences during the relaxation exercise. The leader asks for other ideas on how to relax. Suggestions might include going to a quiet place, lying down, thinking pleasant thoughts, or taking deep breaths.

Members share their illustrations and tell about a place they think is relaxing. It is important to validate each person's experience during this exercise. Some members may not want to close their eyes and can participate with their eyes open. Some members may not be able to visualize a relaxing place. The leader can help focus on a part of the exercise they were able to relate to, such as relaxing the hands by clenching and unclenching or relaxing by taking a deep breath. Members may be able to identify their own relaxation techniques by being asked what they are doing when they feel the most relaxed.

Relaxation

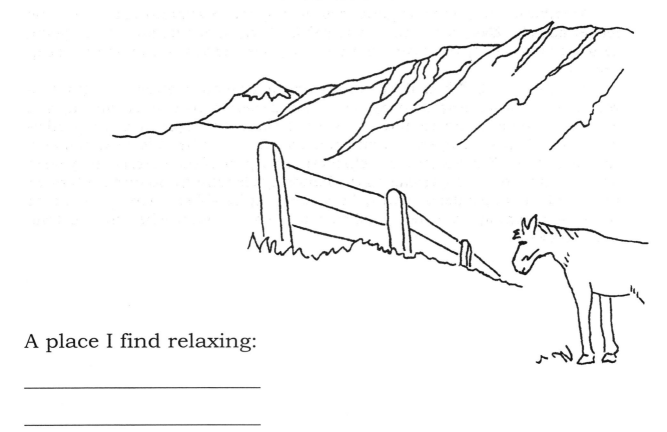

A place I find relaxing:

_____

_____

_____

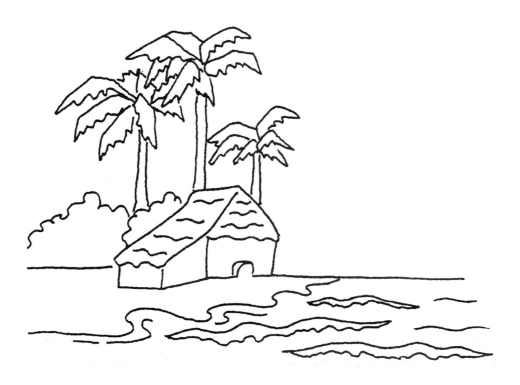

Exercise 16

SURVIVING A HEALTH CRISIS

Purpose:

    1. Emphasize positive coping skills for survival.
    2. Promote group cohesiveness by sharing important personal history.

Materials:

One photocopy of the illustration for each group member; pencils and fine-line colored felt pens or crayons.

Procedure:

    A. While materials are being passed out, members are asked to think about a time they survived a health crisis.
    B. Leader explains that surviving a health crisis makes us aware of our vulnerabilities and also our strengths.
    C Members are asked to draw themselves or someone they know in the hospital scene. If members do not have any experiences with hospitals or ambulances, they are asked to recall some illness they have experienced. Members may color the picture, if they wish.
    D. The sentence fragments are read aloud and members are asked to complete the sentences.

Group Discussion:

    Members share their illustrations and tell about when they themselves or someone they know survived a health crisis. Members are asked to tell what helped them to survive the crisis.

    This exercise helps to promote empathy and understanding for the hardships of others as well as reminding members of strengths they have used to survive.

Surviving a Health Crisis

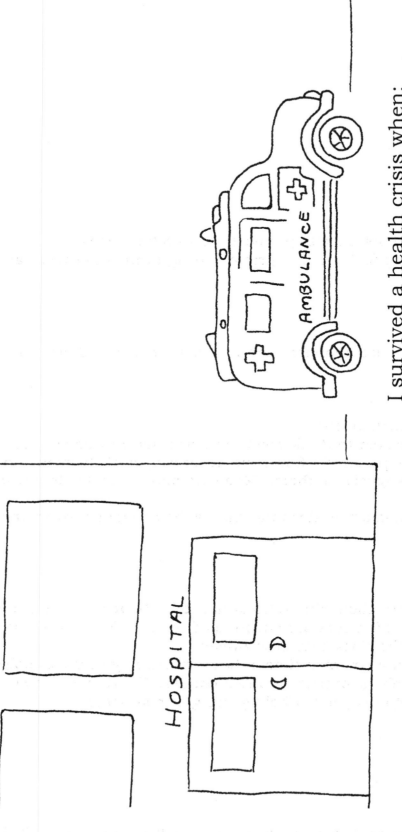

I survived a health crisis when: _____

I coped by: _____

Exercise 17

TIMEPIECES

Purpose:

1. Encourage reminiscence to promote group cohesiveness.
2. Practice sharing feelings in a group setting to increase trust and openness.

Materials:

Photocopy of the illustration for each member; pencils and crayons.

Procedure:

A. Materials are distributed.
B. Members are asked to think about associations they have to the various types of clocks pictured. Some members may wish to draw a watch or clock that was special to them. Members may color the drawings if they wish.
C. Members are asked to write in the blanks their best and worst times of the day.

Group Discussion:

Members share their illustrations and tell about their best and worst times of the day. Members are encouraged to reminisce about the various clocks shown or the clock they have drawn.

Sharing about a common theme that is not highly personal helps members to develop feelings of trust and relatedness. Sharing about worst times of the day can help to open up feelings for group support.

Timepieces

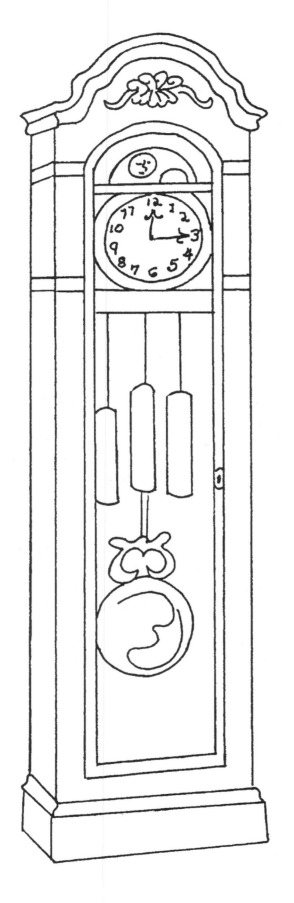

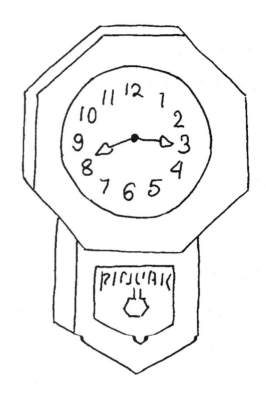

My best time of day: _____

_____

_____

_____

My worst time of day: _____

_____

_____

_____

Exercise 18

WATCH OUT!

Purpose:

1. Share about fears and apprehensions.
2. Promote positive coping techniques to deal with fear.

Materials:

One photocopy of the illustration for each member; pencils and crayons.

Procedure:

A. Materials are distributed. The leader asks members what the people in the picture could be seeing and what they might be feeling.
B. Members are asked to write or draw something that could cause the reactions of the people in the picture, and to write something that causes them to feel fear. Members may color the picture, if they wish.

Group Discussion:

Members share their illustrations and ideas. The leader asks members if they have experienced the feelings depicted in the illustration. Members are encouraged to tell about specific instances of apprehension or fear. The leader asks members to tell how they would cope with the situations described.

This exercise encourages expression of common fears and worries. Members may feel less isolated with their fears and learn new ways to cope.

Watch Out!

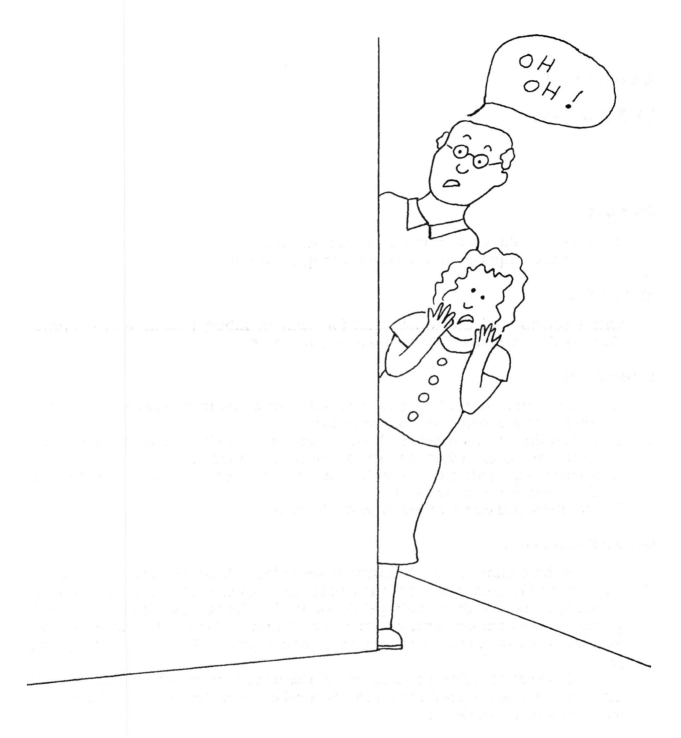

I feel upset when I see: _____

_____

_____

Exercise 19

LETTING GO

Purpose:

1. Allow ventilation of hurts and frustrations.
2. Increase empathy and understanding of others.

Materials:

One photocopy of the illustration for each member; pencils and crayons. *Optional:* blue posterboard, scissors, and glue.

Procedure:

A. While materials are being handed out, group members are asked to think about old resentments they may have.
B. The leader or a member reads the caption on the photocopy. Members are asked to explain what they think the caption means.
C. Members are asked to list in the blanks one or more hurts or resentments they would like to be rid of.
D. Members are encouraged to color the balloon.

Group Discussion:

Members share their illustrations and ideas. Members are asked to tell what makes it hard to let go of their particular resentment, and whether they would feel better if they could get rid of it. The leader asks if anyone in the group can remember getting over a resentment. Those who can share an example are asked to describe how they accomplished letting go and moving on.

This exercise helps focus on one of the important psychological tasks of later life: to work toward resolution of conflicts in order to reduce feelings of worthlessness and despair.

Variation:

The colored balloons can be cut out and glued onto blue posterboard with a copy of the caption as a title.

Letting Go

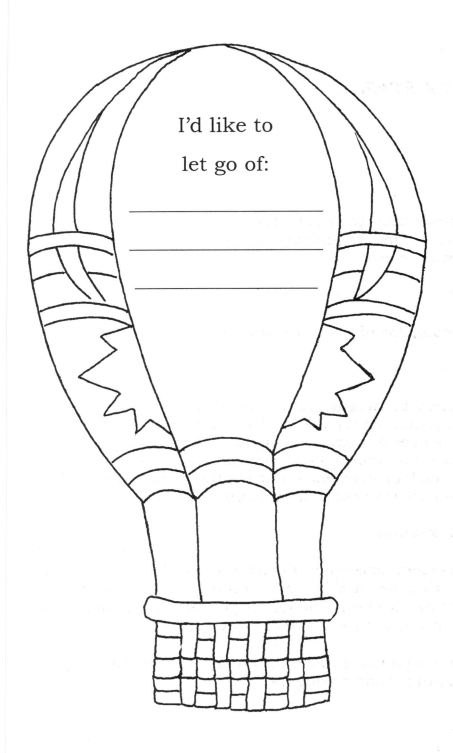

I'd like to

let go of:

_____

_____

_____

Letting go of resentments lightens the heart
and frees the spirit.

Exercise 20

BLOOM WHERE YOU ARE PLANTED

Purpose:

1. Stimulate creative expression and ventilation of feelings.
2. Encourage healthy coping skills.

Materials:

One photocopy of the illustration for each group member; crayons or colored felt pens.

Procedure:

A. Materials are distributed. Group members are asked to explain the meaning of the phrase "Bloom where you are planted."
B. Members are instructed to finish the illustration of flowers in the pot and color their picture.

Group Discussion:

Members share their illustrations and tell why a certain flower or color was chosen. The leader clarifies the meaning of the caption by explaining that the saying "Bloom where you are planted" can mean to make the best of a situation. Members are asked to think of difficult times in their lives when it was hard to make the best of things; for example, a bad work situation or a difficult relationship.

Members are asked to describe how they coped, what helped them to survive, and what they learned from the experience.

Reviewing previous coping skills helps members to stay in touch with personal strengths.

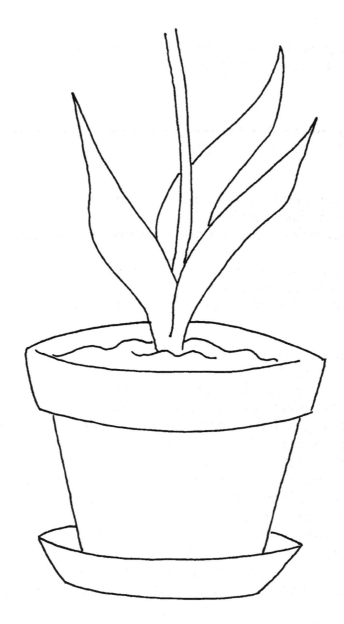

Bloom Where You Are Planted

Exercise 21

MAKING NEW GOALS

Purpose:

1. Encourage positive goal formation to instill hope.
2. Increase awareness of personal needs.

Materials:

One photocopy of the illustration for each member; pencils and crayons.

Procedure:

A. Materials are passed out and the leader points out that making positive goals is psychologically healthy.
B. Members are asked to think about realistic goals that might improve their life.
C. The statements are read aloud and members are asked to complete the sentences with their goals.
D. Members may color the illustration and draw pictures to represent their goals.

Group Discussion:

Members are asked to share memories and associations triggered by the illustration. The leader asks members to share how they have celebrated the New Year and whether they have made New Year's resolutions.

The leader explains that it is important to make resolutions or set goals throughout the year and throughout life. Members are asked to give examples of realistic, positive goals. Suggestions might include smiling more often, remembering to express appreciation to others, making a new acquaintance, or participating in more activities.

Members share their illustrations and goals. They are asked to explain how they might go about achieving their goals.

This exercise is helpful in stimulating interest in setting realistic goals and raising awareness of remaining areas of choice in the members' lives.

Making New Goals

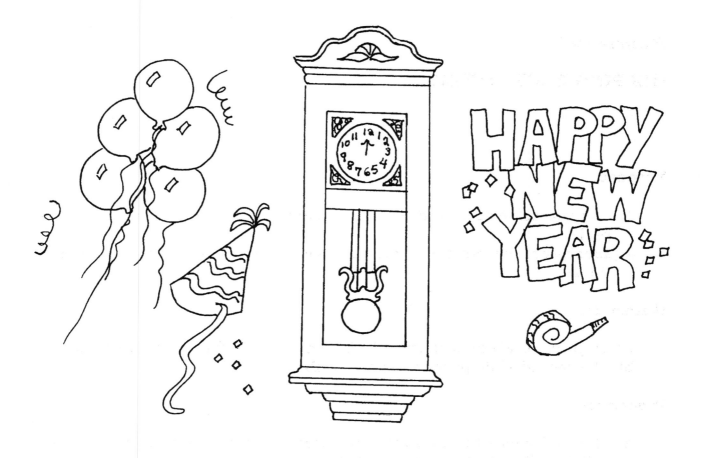

I would like to do more: _____

_____

_____

I would like to do less: _____

_____

_____

A goal for next week: _____

_____

_____

Exercise 22

HELPING EACH OTHER

Purpose:

1. Increase self-esteem and feelings of belonging by participation in a group project.
2. Emphasize the value of altruistic behavior which enhances positive self-image.

Materials:

Large piece of white posterboard; fine-line colored felt pens. **Optional:** a blank sheet of white paper for each member.

Procedure:

A. The leader tells the group that members are going to make a poster together to illustrate helpful attitudes.
B. The leader explains that being helpful is not only beneficial to others but also helps people to feel better about themselves.
C. The group is asked to share ideas on how they can be helpful to others.
D. Each group member selects a colored fine-line felt pen to be used on the poster. It is best to omit yellow because it does not show up well on white posterboard.
E. The leader uses the colored pen chosen by the group member to draw around one hand of the member, placing the palm on the edge of the posterboard with the fingers pointing toward the middle (see example on p. 53). A large piece of posterboard accomodates 8 to 10 outlines of hands with some overlapping of the fingers.
F. Members are asked to write their names on the outline of their hand in the same color used to draw around the hand.
G. The leader selects a colored felt pen and writes "Helping Hands" in large letters in the middle of the poster.

Group Discussion:

The leader encourages members to tell stories about how they have helped someone in the past or present. Members may also tell about special times when they received help. This exercise focuses on positive actions of self and others to increase trust and cooperation.

Variation:

This exercise can be done individually by drawing around members' hands on separate pieces of paper.

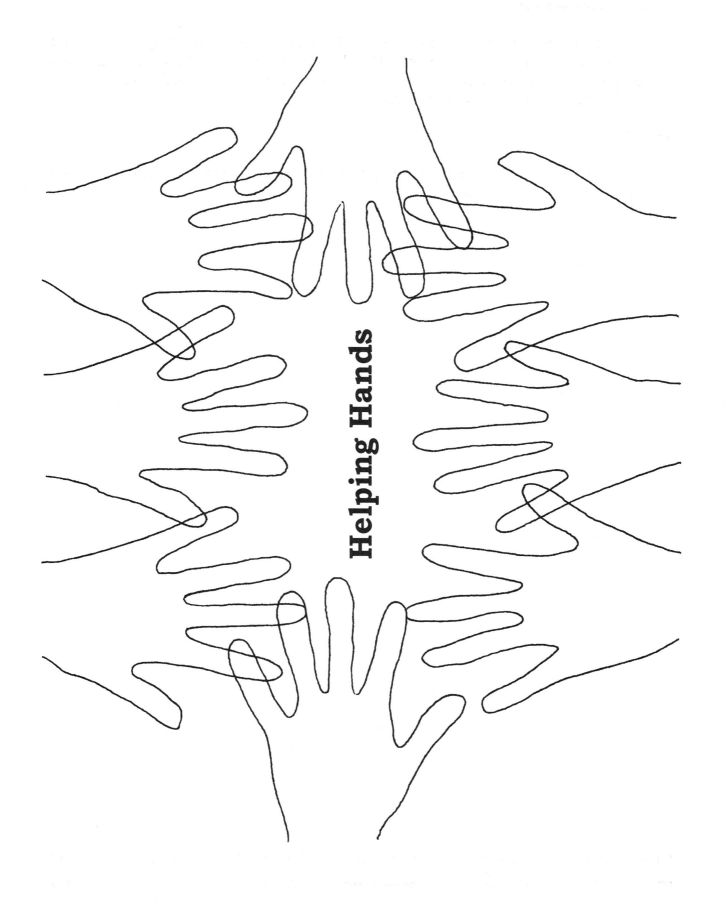

Exercise 23

MEMORIES OF FATHER

Purpose:

1. Increase understanding of self and others by sharing feelings about family.
2. Promote resolution of past emotional issues.

Materials:

One photocopy of the illustration for each member; pencils or fine-line colored felt pens.

Procedure:

A. Members are asked to recall memories of their father or a father figure in their lives.
B. Materials are distributed and members are encouraged to draw a picture of their father in the frame.
C. The sentence fragments are read aloud and members are instructed to fill in responses.

Group Discussion:

Members share their illustrations and sentences. Validation of feelings is very important in this exercise. Some members may express feelings of loss or unresolved grief about their father. Other members may reveal unpleasant memories or disappointments. In these cases, members can be encouraged to share how they survived and what they did to make up for their fathers' deficits. Members may also be encouraged to tell how their feelings about their father have changed over time.

Memories of Father

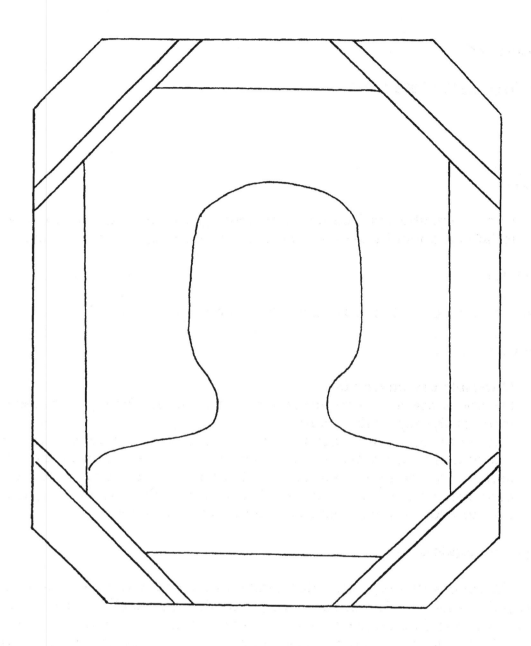

My father was good at: _____

I liked it when he: _____

Sometimes I wished he would: _____

If I could talk to him today, I'd tell him: _____

_____

Exercise 24

HOW DO YOU FEEL?

Purpose:

1. Encourage sharing feelings to promote group empathy and support.
2. Relate emotional states to stressors in order to enhance coping abilities.

Materials:

One photocopy of the illustration for each member; pencils.

Procedure:

A. Materials are passed out.
B. Members are asked to guess what feelings are being expressed on the faces at the top of the exercise.
C. The situations under the blank faces are read out loud. Members are instructed to draw faces that reflect their own feelings in the situations listed. The leader emphasizes that the illustrated faces at the top of the page can be used as examples, but that members are free to draw their own interpretations of expressions on the blank faces.

Group Discussion:

Members display their illustrations and share their feelings about the situations listed. The group leader explains that feelings are neither good nor bad, but that people have choices about how to handle their feelings.

Members are asked for suggestions on how to cope with problematic situations such as those listed. By sharing ideas in a group setting, members may learn new coping strategies.

How Do You Feel?

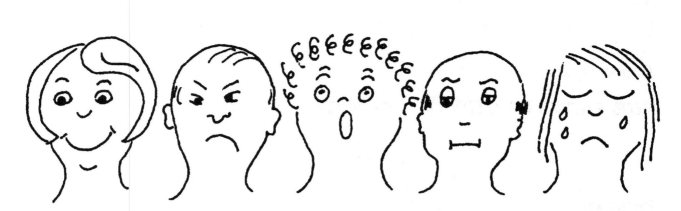

Examples

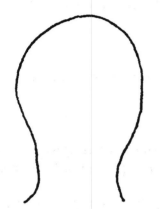

When I
Wake Up

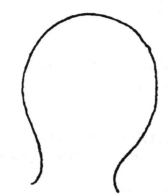

When Someone
Visits

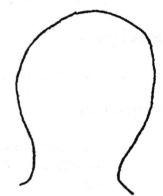

At Mealtime

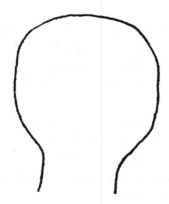

When People
Argue

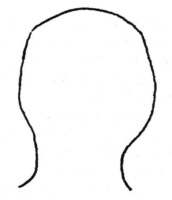

When I
See the
Doctor

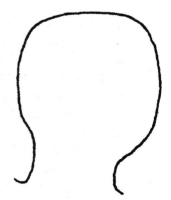

When I
Go to Bed

Exercise 25

THE FABLE OF THE TWO GOATS

Purpose:

1. Allow ventilation of frustrations regarding self and others.
2. Promote positive coping strategies to deal with interpersonal stresses.

Materials:

One photocopy of the illustration for each member; pencils and crayons.

Procedure:

A. The leader explains that fables are stories that are passed from generation to generation because they illustrate truths about people that last over time.
B. Materials are passed out and the leader or a member reads the story (Aesop's Fable) of the two goats out loud.
C. Members are asked to tell what they think the story means.
D. Members may color the picture if they wish.

Group Discussion:

Members share their illustrations and are asked to tell about stubborn individuals they have encountered in their lives. The leader asks members what they did to cope with the stubborn behavior. The leader validates feelings of frustration expressed by the members and acknowledges the difficulty of altering beliefs and behavior.

Members are asked if they have experienced feeling stubborn themselves about an issue and what led up to this feeling. The leader asks if there is a difference between being stubborn and holding one's ground. The leader points out that holding one's ground can be a beneficial decision if it helps to prevent self-defeating behavior such as alcohol or drug abuse.

The Fable of
The Two Goats

Once upon a time two proud goats stared at each other from opposite cliffs of a high mountain range. Between the cliffs lay a deep, rocky valley with a raging river at the bottom. The only bridge across the river was a fallen tree so narrow that only one goat could pass at a time. Both stubborn goats felt they had the right to cross the river first, and each immediately proceeded to walk across the slender log. The two goats met head to head in the middle of the bridge. Neither goat would give way to the other, and, finally, both goats fell headlong into the raging river below.

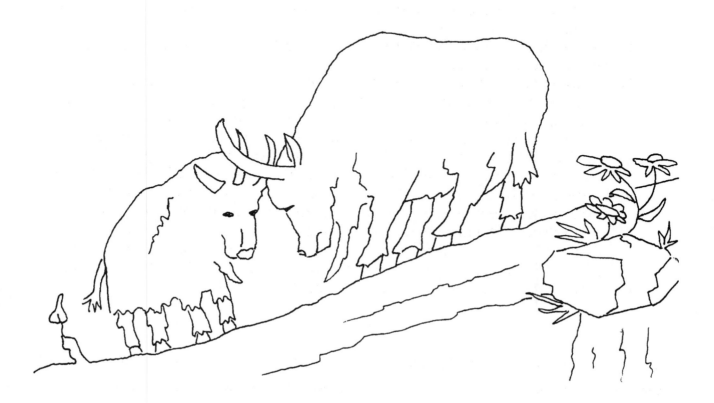

Exercise 26

THINKING AND FEELING

Purpose:

1. Raise awareness of how thoughts affect feelings.
2. Share feelings to increase group cohesion.

Materials:

One photocopy of the illustration for each member; pencils and fine-line colored felt pens or crayons.

Procedure:

A. Materials are distributed and the leader or a member reads the caption aloud.
B. Members are asked to explain the meaning of the saying "You can't control how other people think and feel, but you can often choose your own thoughts and attitudes."
C. The leader points out that the way you think about a situation affects how you feel about the situation.
D. As an example of how a person's choice of thoughts affects feelings, members are asked to think about annoying dinner partners who may be complaining, rude, or unmannerly. Members are asked how they feel about food when they think about this subject. Members are then asked to think about food at a meal they enjoy, specifically recalling how the food looks and what it tastes like. Members are asked how they feel about these thoughts. The leader points out that how a person feels about dinner is influenced by the kind of thoughts the person is having about the experience and what aspects of the meal the person is focusing on.
E. Members are asked to complete the sentences in the illustration and draw a face that shows how the thought makes them feel. Members may draw food on the plate and color the picture if they wish.

Group Discussion:

Members share their illustrations and responses. The leader asks members to share other examples of how thoughts affect feelings. Members are asked to tell about times when it is hard to change one's thoughts. The leader should validate and acknowledge members' feelings. The leader should keep in mind that members who hear voices or have mood disorders may experience times when they cannot choose their thoughts. The leader encourages hope by giving examples of times when the member was able to choose his or her way of thinking. For example, the leader might ask if the member chose to cooperate with bathing this week, or if the member chose to refuse and dwell on how much work it is to get undressed and ready for bath time.

This exercise helps members to realize that they can improve their own mood by choosing to think of unpleasant events in a different way. The idea of changing one's own mood is particularly empowering to elder group members because, in many ways, their choices in life have become very restricted.

Thinking and Feeling

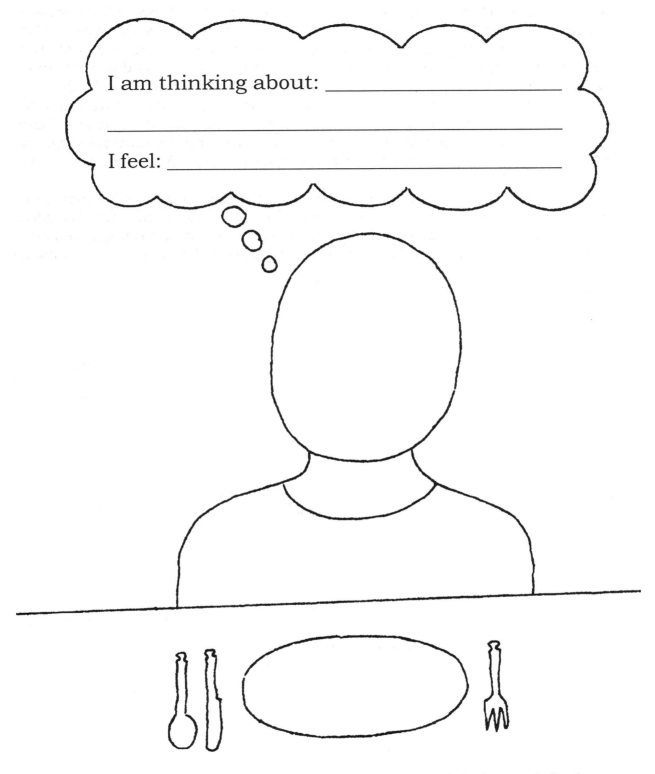

I am thinking about: _____

_____

I feel: _____

You can't control how other people think and feel,
but you can often choose your own thoughts and attitudes.

Exercise 27

HUMOROUS HALLOWEEN STORY

Purpose:

1. Stimulate imagination and sense of humor.
2. Promote group cohesion by cooperating in story creation.

Materials:

A pencil and one photocopy of the exercise and story for the leader.

Procedure:

A. The leader explains that the group is going to make up a Halloween story together.
B. The leader goes around the group circle asking for contributions one at a time to fill in the blanks on the top of the group leader's worksheet (see p. 66).
C. The group leader then reads the story on the bottom of the group leader's worksheet (p. 66), filling in the blanks with the words supplied by the members.

Group Discussion:

Members share their reactions to the story and tell whether they ever played a Halloween trick on someone. Members are asked to share other memories about Halloween, such as experiences of "trick-or-treating" and wearing costumes. Members who did not celebrate Halloween are asked how they felt about not being included.

Most group members enjoy participating in creating a humorous story. Sharing humor helps to increase a sense of well-being and a feeling of belonging.

Group Leader's Worksheet
for Humorous Halloween Story

1. A pet: _____

2. A vegetable: _____

3. Some type of candy: _____

4. A reptile: _____

5. A spice: _____

6. A jungle animal: _____

7. A color: _____

8. A room in the house: _____

9. A farm animal sound: _____

10. A piece of furniture: _____

- -

THE LITTLE WITCH

One Halloween the littlest witch decided to play a trick on her pet _____. She made a potion out of cold
1
_____, gooey _____, ground up
2   3
_____, and lots of _____. She
4   5
stirred the potion in a big black pot over the fire. When it was ready, she fed it to her pet _____. Her pet
1
_____ turned into a _____ with
1   6
_____ horns. It chased the little witch all around
7
the _____, crying loudly _____!
8   9
_____! The little witch hid under the
9
_____ and missed Halloween altogether. At mid-
10
night, the spell was broken and the little witch's pet returned to normal. She never played a Halloween trick on her pet again.

Exercise 28

HOW DO YOU DO?

Purpose:

1. Promote self-disclosure to increase positive sense of self.
2. Enhance relatedness by increasing awareness of others.

Materials:

One photocopy of the illustration for each member; pencils, crayons, or fine-line colored felt pens.

Procedure:

A. Materials are distributed and the leader explains that the group is going to do an introduction exercise to get to know each other better.

B. Members are instructed to fill in the blanks on the worksheet. A volunteer is selected to help members who do not write, so that each group member has a completed worksheet.

Group Discussion:

Members share their introductions. After each presentation, the member being introduced selects another group member to ask two questions about the material presented in the introduction. A different member is selected each time so that everyone has an opportunity to ask questions.

This exercise helps to reduce self-absorption and isolation by encouraging interest in others. The exercise enhances identity and encourages good listening skills.

How Do You Do?

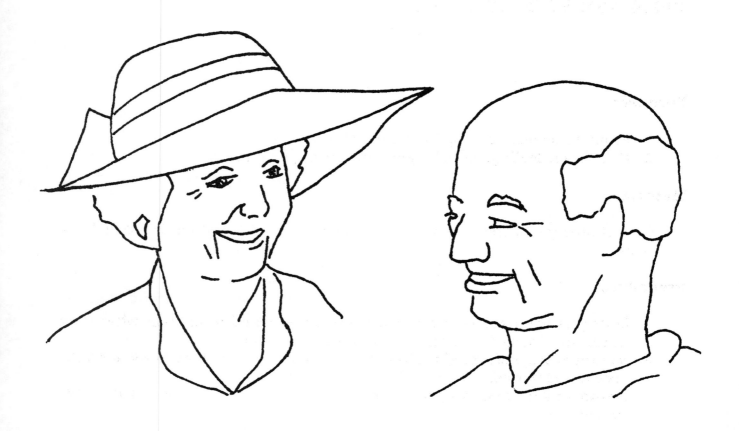

My name is: _____

I grew up in: _____

I enjoy: _____

Today I feel: _____

Exercise 29

TAKE ONE STEP AT A TIME

Purpose:

1. Promote positive coping by instilling hope.
2. Encourage feelings of belonging by sharing memories.

Materials:

One photocopy of the illustration for each member; crayons or colored felt pens.

Procedure:

A. Materials are passed out and members are asked to explain what they think the saying "Take one step at a time" means.
B. Members are instructed to circle or color footwear that they associate with special memories.
C. Members who wish may draw or color a favorite pair of shoes they have owned.

Group Discussion:

Members share their illustrations and memories about the shoes pictured or other special memories about footwear.

The leader asks members to give specific examples of times in their lives when they have needed to "Take one step at a time." Examples might include taking one step at a time to recover from an illness, make a new friend, or handle a problem.

This exercise encourages a hopeful attitude by reminding members to work on problems gradually beginning with small steps.

Take One Step at a Time.

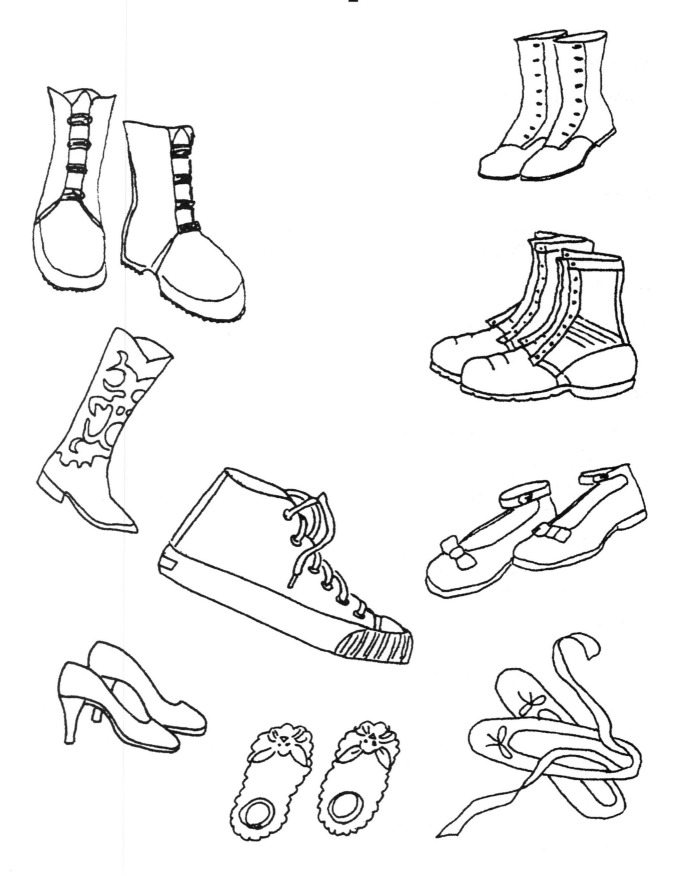

Exercise 30

APPRECIATING DIFFERENCES

Purpose:

1. Increase tolerance of differences in others.
2. Build feelings of group cohesion and cooperation.

Materials:

Photocopies of wildflowers cut apart so that there is at least one flower for each member; one large sheet of green posterboard; fine-line colored felt pens; extra blank paper.

Procedure:

A. The leader explains that the group is going to make a poster together to illustrate the topic "Sharing Our Similarities, and Appreciating Our Differences."
B. Members are asked to explain how the topic could apply to people residing in a group living situation.
C. The pictures of the flowers are shown to the group so that each member can choose a picture to color. Some members may want to draw and color their own flower design.
D. The colored pictures are glued onto the posterboard with the topic "Sharing Our Similarities, and Appreciating Our Differences" as a title.

Group Discussion:

Members are asked to share memories about the various wildflowers pictured and reactions to the finished poster.

The leader points out that it is often easier to "share similarities" than it is to "appreciate differences." The members are asked what some of the differences are among people in a group living situation that are difficult to handle. The leader may ask members for ideas on coping strategies to deal with frustrations that are expressed.

Members in a group living situation are frequently stressed by close contact with persons very different from themselves. Venting feelings and sharing coping strategies helps members to deal more effectively with the daily stresses of group living.

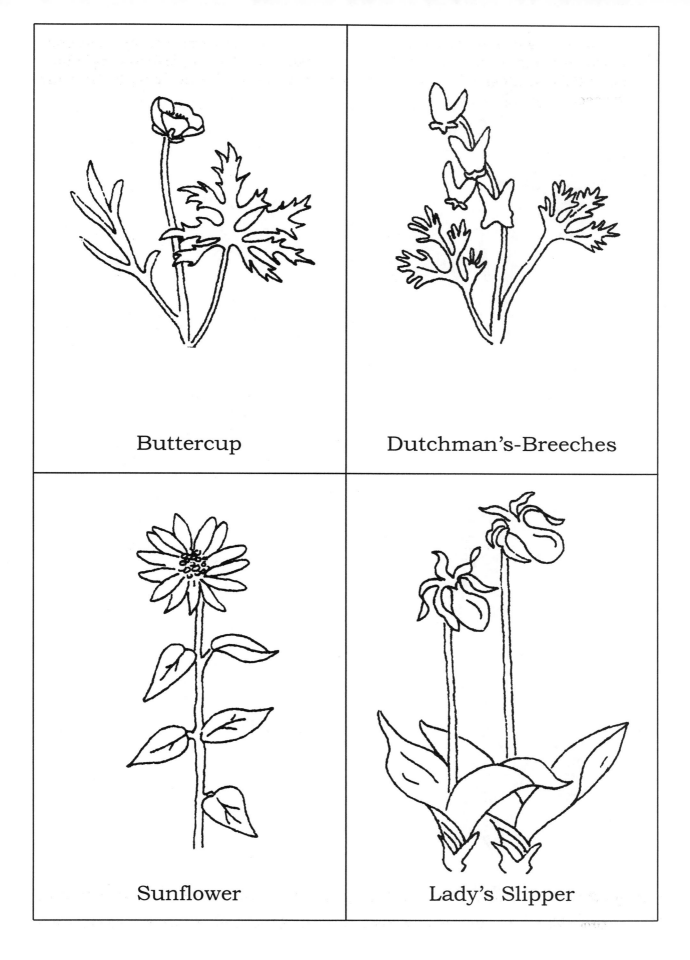

Buttercup

Dutchman's-Breeches

Sunflower

Lady's Slipper

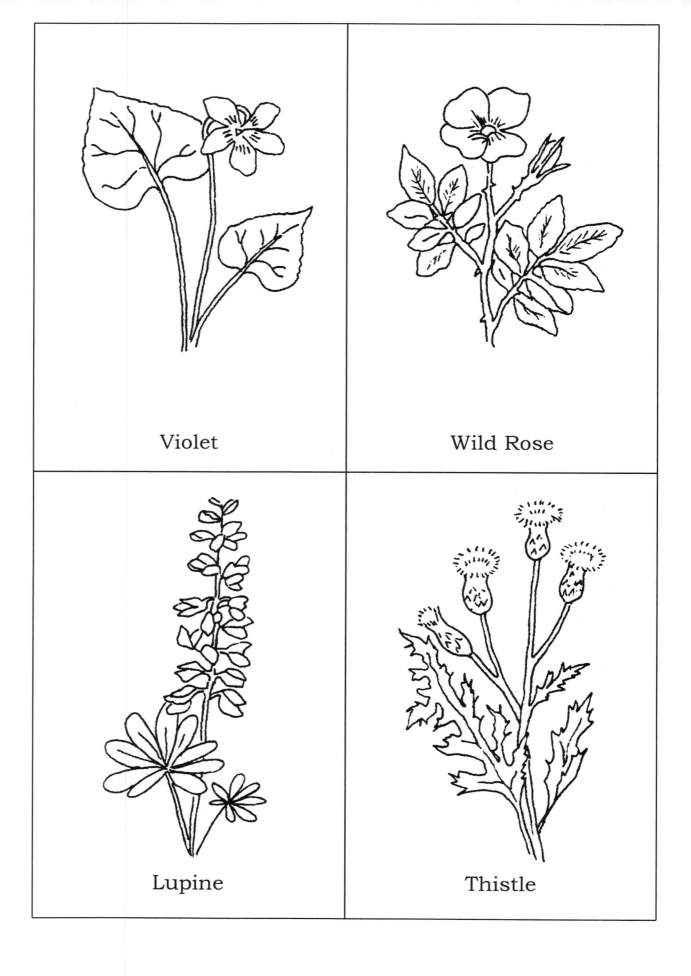

Violet

Wild Rose

Lupine

Thistle

Exercise 31

THE BEST THINGS IN LIFE ARE FREE

Purpose:

1. Encourage positive ideation.
2. Stimulate interest in and appreciation for the environment.

Materials:

One photocopy of the illustration for each member; pencils, colored felt pens, or crayons. ***Optional:*** posterboard, glue, and scissors.

Procedure:

A. While materials are being distributed, group members are asked to think of enjoyable things in life that are free.
B. Members are asked to color the picture and add a flower design if they wish.
C. Members are instructed to list things that are enjoyable and free.

Group Discussion:

Members share their illustrations and lists. The leader encourages expression of as many ideas as possible, making special note of ideas accessible to the group members, such as a friendly greeting, a smile, or a hopeful attitude.

This exercise raises group members' awareness of opportunities for enjoyment that don't cost money. Many elder group members are on a fixed income and appreciate ideas about mood-enhancing experiences that are free.

Variation:

The butterflies can be cut out and glued onto posterboard with the caption "The Best Things in Life Are Free" as a title. The ideas suggested by group members can be written between the butterflies with felt pen.

The Best Things in Life Are Free.

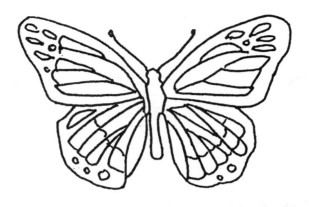

Some things in life that are free:

_____

_____

_____

_____

_____

_____

_____

_____

_____

_____

_____

Exercise 32

HOUSE OF FEARS

Purpose:

1. Encourage cohesion and relatedness by cooperating on a group project.
2. Increase understanding of self and others by sharing memories.

Materials:

One large sheet of orange posterboard, 22" x 28"; one 12" x 18" piece of brown construction paper and one or two 9" x 12" pieces of yellow construction paper; fine-line black felt pens, scissors, and glue stick.

Procedure:

A. The leader explains that the group is going to make a poster of a haunted house.
B. Group leader cuts 2" x 6" triangles out of the top corners of the brown paper to form a roof line for a house (see illustration of house on page 79). The leader folds a 9" x 12" piece of yellow construction paper into eighths and cuts on the folds to form eight rectangles for windows and a door.
C. Each group member is given one of the small yellow rectangles and asked to draw a Halloween design on it with a black felt pen. Members who like to draw are asked to help members who do not draw. Suggestions for designs might include pumpkins, ghosts, witches, skeletons, and so forth. One rectangle is chosen for the front door.
D. The leader glues the brown house onto the orange posterboard and glues on the "windows" and "door." Black grill-work on the rooftop and a few bats in the sky can be added with black felt pens. The poster is labeled "House of Fears" with a black felt pen.

Group Discussion:

Members are asked to share Halloween memories and fears. The leader asks if members ever thought a house was haunted and whether they believe in ghosts, or whether they were afraid of the dark.

Members share feelings and reactions to seeing their artwork combined into a group poster.

Contributing to a creative group project enhances a sense of belonging and increases self-esteem. Sharing childhood fears and fantasies promotes group cohesion.

Variation:

Each member is given a copy of the illustration and asked to draw or write fears in the window spaces.

House of Fears

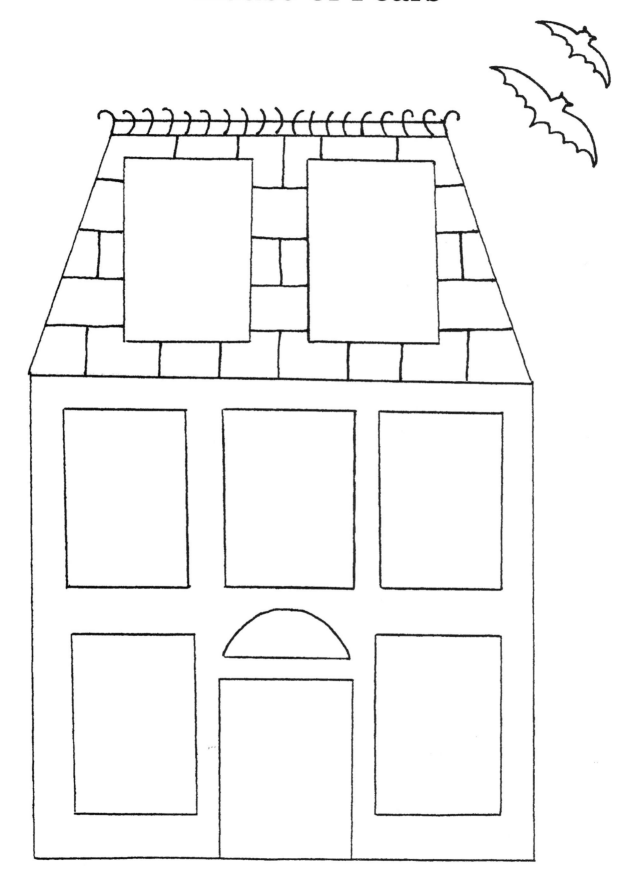

Exercise 33

THANKSGIVING CARDS

Purpose:

1. Increase awareness of the feelings of others.
2. Build feelings of community and group cohesion.

Materials:

One photocopy of the illustration for each group member; colored fine-line felt pens; small slips of paper and a hat or box.

Procedure:

A. While materials are being passed out, the leader explains that the photocopy is a Thanksgiving card.
B. Members are instructed to fold the photocopy in half and then in half again to form a card.
C. The leader writes each member's name on a small piece of paper and puts the name in a hat.
D. Each member draws a name from the hat and writes this name on the card.
E. Members are asked to identify the pictures on the front and back of the card. The leader points out that the food items on the back of the card are often pictured in cornucopias.
F. Members are encouraged to draw and color items in the cornucopia to complete the picture.
G. Members are asked to sign their name inside the card. They may also write a Thanksgiving message if they wish.

Group Discussion:

Members exchange cards and share the card they received, displaying the card and telling who gave them the card. Members share feelings and reactions to making and receiving handmade cards. The leader points out that it is not always necessary to buy an expensive card to convey a thoughtful message.

This group exercise is helpful in building feelings of belonging and inclusion.

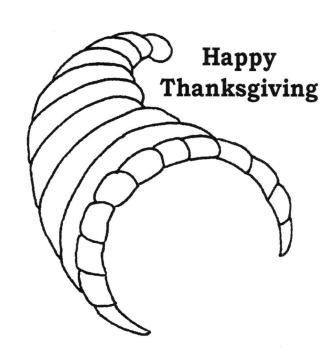

Happy
Thanksgiving

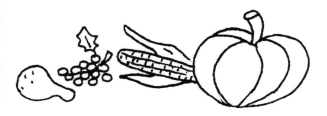

Exercise 34

CHANGES IN OUR LIVES

Purpose:

1. Share feelings about changes in life.
2. Encourage positive attitudes about change.

Materials:

One photocopy of the illustration for each member; fine-line colored felt pens. *Optional:* posterboard to make a group collage.

Procedure:

A. As materials are being distributed, members are asked to think about changes in their lives.
B. The leader or a group member reads the caption on the photocopy. Members are asked to explain what they think the saying means.
C. Members are asked to color fall leaves on the trees to represent changes in nature.

Group Discussion:

The leader explains that many people resist change because they are afraid of the unknown, but changes can sometimes lead to new opportunities such as losing a job and finding a better one or moving to a different location and meeting new friends. Members are asked to tell about changes in their lives that have led to new opportunities. Discussion topics might include moving to a new place, changing jobs, improvements in health care, or changes in family structure. Members are asked to tell about attitudes that help a person adapt to change, such as flexibility, open-mindedness, and willingness to try new experiences.

Many changes in life are unavoidable. Sharing feelings about change and ways to adjust to new circumstances helps members to strengthen their abilities to cope with changes in their lives.

Variation:

A group poster can be made by cutting a rectangle around each tree to remove excess border and gluing the tree designs to colored posterboard. A copy of the caption can be used as a title for the poster.

Members often experience pride and increased self-esteem from seeing their artwork combined into a group poster.

Changes in Our Lives

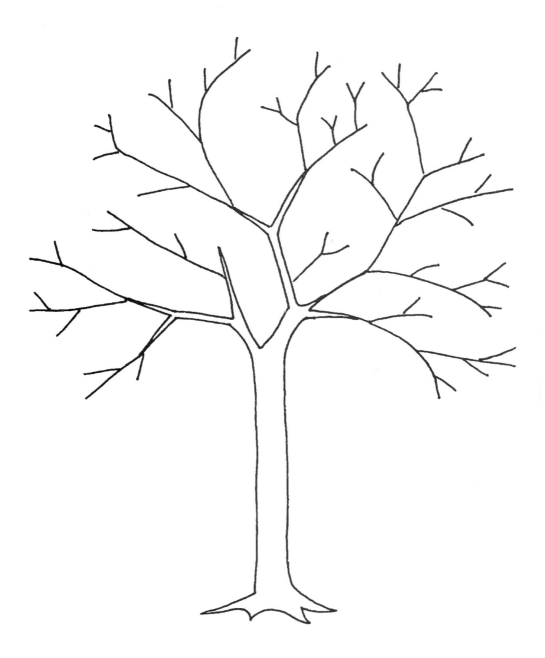

Changes in our lives
Like changes in the seasons
Bring new challenges
And opportunities for growth.

Exercise 35

LET'S PRESERVE

Purpose:

1. Increase relatedness by sharing memories in a nonthreatening format.
2. Stimulate positive cognition and goal formation.

Materials:

One photocopy of the illustration for each member; crayons and pencils.

Procedure:

A. Materials are passed out and group members are encouraged to share memories of canning, preserving, or other methods of food preservation.
B. Members are asked to describe the contents of the first jar and fill in the label if they wish.
C. The leader points out that the idea of preserving can be applied to saving the environment. Members are asked to give ideas regarding natural resources that need preservation efforts.
D. Members are asked to write in or draw and color items for preserving in the empty jar. Drawings may depict actual food items or environmental concerns. Other ideas can be listed on the blank lines.

Group Discussion:

Members share their illustrations and ideas. Members are asked to share memories of canning and food preservation. Topics of discussion might include pickling, use of smokehouses, and fruit cellars.

Members are encouraged to explore whether their residence supports recycling efforts and find out ways they can help.

This exercise encourages reminiscence as well as stimulating interest in current topics of concern about environmental issues. Encouraging interest in current affairs helps to increase motivation and interest in living.

Let's Preserve

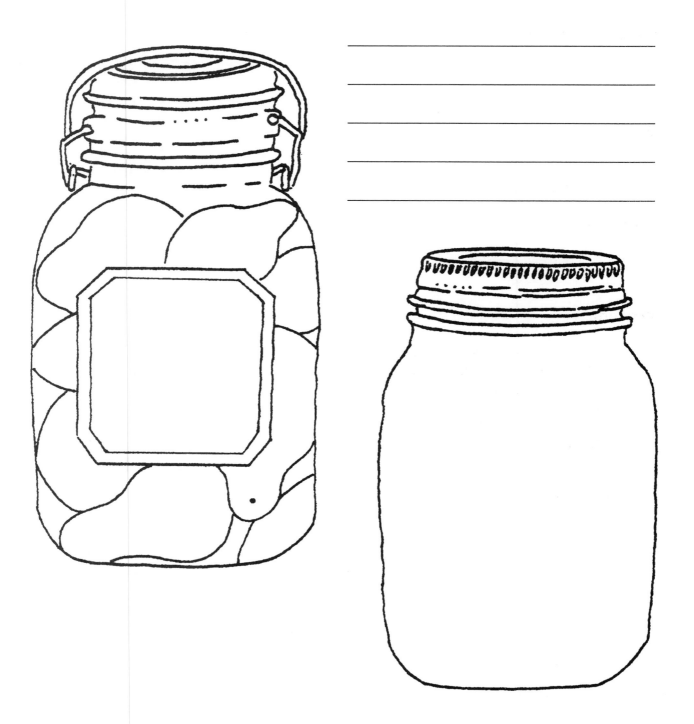

Exercise 36

COW KNOW-HOW

Purpose:

1. Share positive coping skills in a humorous, nonthreatening format.
2. Promote self-disclosure and greater awareness of others.

Materials:

One photocopy of the illustration for each group member; pencils and crayons.

Procedure:

A. Materials are distributed.
B. Members go around the circle taking turns reading lines in the "Cow Know-How" worksheet.
C. Members check boxes opposite statements that have been addressed to themselves or others in their childhood.
D. Members may color the picture if they wish and add other farm details to the picture.

Group Discussion:

Members share their illustrations and tell why they checked certain statements. The leader explains that early family messages affect a person's self-image. Members discuss which sayings are helpful and which should be replaced with more positive self-statements.

Members are asked to add to the list other negative or positive messages from childhood that had an impact on their self-image.

This exercise encourages self-revelation and opens the participants to feedback which may help to form a more positive self-image.

Cow Know-How

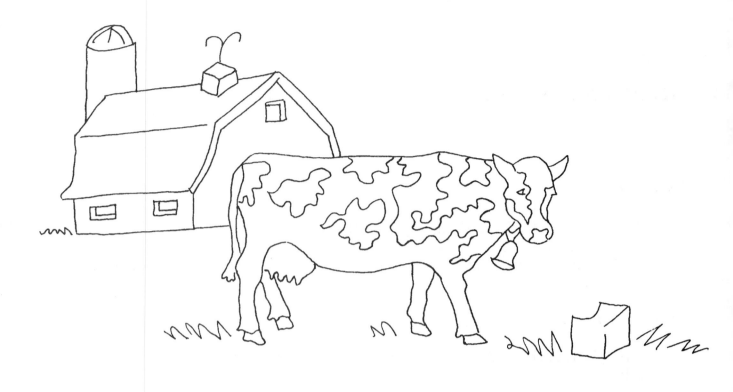

☐ The grass is greener on the other side.

☐ Don't cry over spilled milk.

☐ Children are to be seen and not herd.

☐ Take the bull by the horns.

☐ Don't be Bossy!

☐ Clumsy as a bull in a china closet.

☐ Cow-nt your blessings.

☐ Don't go to bed in an angry moo-d.

Exercise 37

SWEET MEMORIES

Purpose:

1. Share memories and feelings about a common subject to enhance feelings of belonging.
2. Promote group support for coping with dietary restrictions and limitations.

Materials:

One photocopy of the illustration for each group member; crayons and pencils.

Procedure:

A. As materials are being passed out, members are asked to think about experiences they have had with ice cream parlors and soda fountains.
B. The leader encourages members to write their favorite ice cream treat in the blank, draw the treat, and color the pictures.

Group Discussion:

Members share memories about the illustration, ice cream parlors, and soda fountains. Each member shows his or her illustration and tells about a favorite ice cream treat. Reminiscing about a nonthreatening subject helps to build group cohesion.

The leader asks if any members have dietary limitations for ice cream, sweets, or other foods. Members who have special dietary needs are asked to tell about their diets and how they feel about the restrictions.

Group support and encouragement is offered to members who express frustrations or resentments about their diets. Sharing feelings about dietary restrictions helps members to handle frustration and learn new ways to cope.

Sweet Memories

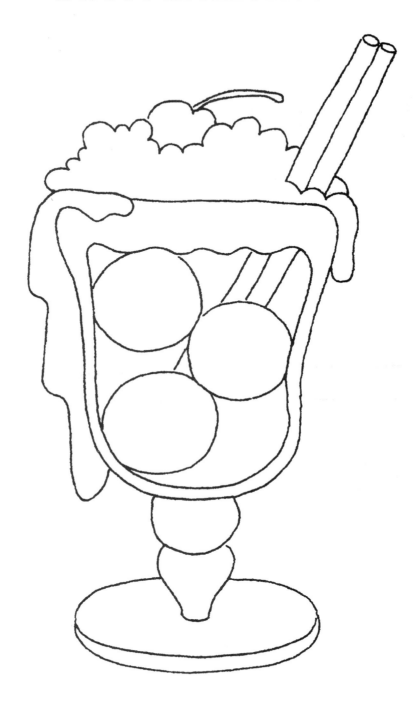

My favorite ice cream treat: _____

_____

Exercise 38

FEELING TRAPPED

Purpose:

1. Open up feelings of frustration for group support.
2. Share ideas on ways to overcome feelings of isolation and entrapment.

Materials:

One photocopy of the illustration for each member; pencils and crayons.

Procedure:

A. Photocopies are distributed and members are asked to identify the picture.
B. The leader or a member describes how a minnow bucket is used to trap minnows which are then used as bait for fishing.
C. Members are asked to think about times in their lives when they have felt trapped and how they handled the situation.
D. Members are asked to complete the sentences below the picture. Members may color the illustration if they wish.

Group Discussion:

Members share their sentences about feeling trapped and describe how they handled the situation. The group leader encourages support by acknowledging that everyone has felt trapped at some time in their lives.

Some members may feel trapped in their present living situation. Ideas for coping and suggestions for feeling less confined are elicited from the group. Sharing frustrations and discussing coping techniques reduces feelings of isolation and helplessness.

Members are asked to share memories about using a minnow bucket or other fishing experiences. Reminiscing about a common subject builds feelings of relatedness and belonging.

Feeling Trapped

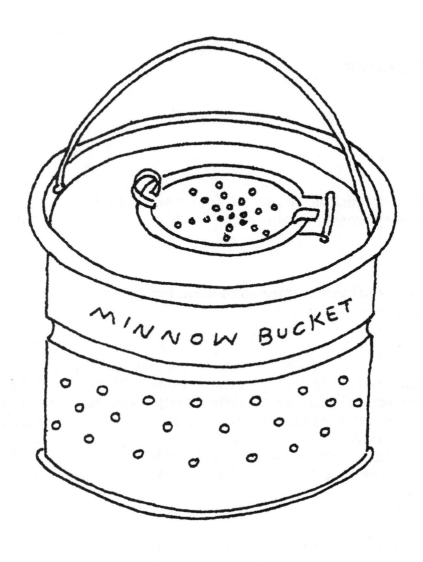

I felt trapped when: _____

_____

_____

I handled the situation by: _____

_____

_____

Exercise 39

HOLIDAY LETTER

Purpose:

1. Improve relatedness by increasing communication.
2. Expand awareness of others.

Materials:

One photocopy of the letter for each member; pencils and crayons. ***Optional:*** slips of paper and a hat or box.

Procedure:

A. Materials are distributed and the sentence fragments are read aloud.
B. Members are asked to write "Dear Group" and fill in the blanks in the rest of the letter. If needed, help is given so that all group members can complete the letter.
C. Members are encouraged to color the picture and add additional holiday designs to the border of the letter if they wish.

Group Discussion:

Members present their illustrations and read their letters to the group. The leader asks group members to share about other special holiday memories.

This exercise is effective in promoting group cohesiveness and encouraging shy members to open up.

Variation:

Members may draw each other's names from a hat and write a letter to the member whose name was drawn. In this variation make sure adequate help and supervision are provided for the letter writing so that each member receives a completed, appropriate holiday letter.

Holiday Letter

Dear _____ ,

I remember celebrating the holidays by: _____

_____

_____

I especially liked: _____

_____

For a holiday dinner we often had: _____

_____

I hope your holiday is filled with: _____

_____

Don't forget to: _____

_____

_____

Warm holiday wishes from

_____

Exercise 40

MEMORIES OF MOTHER

Purpose:

1. Increase understanding of self and others by sharing feelings about family.
2. Work through unfinished or unresolved feelings about mother or mother figure.

Materials:

One photocopy of the illustration for each member; pencils and fine-line colored felt pens.

Procedure:

A. Members are asked to think about their mother or a mother figure in their lives.
B. Materials are distributed and the sentence fragments are read aloud.
C. Members are asked to complete the sentences.
D. The leader encourages members to draw and color a picture of their mother or a mother figure in the frame.

Group Discussion:

Members share their pictures and feelings about mother. The leader asks members to share how they are similar to or different from their mother. If a group member had no mother figure, that member may share ideas on the mother he or she would like to have had.

This exercise is effective in helping members gain perspective on their relationship with their mother. Members who vent feelings of disappointment about their mothers may be asked to share how they made up for their mothers' deficiencies and what coping skills they used to survive.

Memories of Mother

My mother was good at: _____

I liked it when she: _____

Sometimes I wished she would: _____

If I could talk to her today, I'd tell her: _____

_____

Exercise 41

SHARING TRAVELS

Purpose:

1. Promote self-disclosure to enhance identity and relatedness.
2. Increase awareness of common experiences to increase understanding of others.

Materials:

One copy of the photocopy of the illustration for each member; crayons.

Procedure:

A. Photocopies of the illustration and crayons are passed out to the members.
B. Group leader encourages members to identify points of interest shown on the map and to share about those they have visited or lived near.
C. Members may color in areas of special interest.

Group Discussion:

Members are asked to share about a special vacation or other travel experience they have had or would like to have had.

The leader asks members how they felt about family vacations when they were growing up. Members are asked to describe their role in the family vacation. Members who did not take family vacations are asked to tell what they would like to have done for a vacation. Members are asked to tell whether they planned similar or different vacations later in life.

By sharing about vacations and travel, members may discover common interests and experiences. Sharing personal history of this nature enhances identity and promotes reminiscence.

Sharing Travels

Exercise 42

A STITCH IN TIME SAVES NINE

Purpose:

1. Encourage positive coping strategies by increasing insight about problem solving.
2. Promote feelings of belonging by sharing memories.

Materials:

One photocopy of the illustration for each member; pencils and crayons.

Procedure:

A. Materials are distributed and members are asked to identify the picture.
B. The sentence fragments are read aloud and members are asked to write in their responses.
C. Members are asked to draw and color something they made or something made for them. If the item is clothing, it can be drawn on the hanger.

Group Discussion:

The leader asks members to share their memories and associations to the illustration of the treadle sewing machine or to other kinds of sewing machines. Sharing memories promotes group cohesiveness.

Members share their drawings and sentences.

The leader asks members to tell how they feel about living in a more mechanized world where handiwork is less prevalent than in the past.

Members are asked to tell the meaning of the saying "A stitch in time saves nine." The leader explains that the saying can mean to take care of a problem before it grows into a bigger problem. The leader asks group members to give examples from their own lives. Examples might include taking care of a health problem before it worsens or communicating about a problem to prevent a fight. This exercise raises awareness about the importance of taking care of health and other problems before they become much worse.

A Stitch in Time Saves Nine

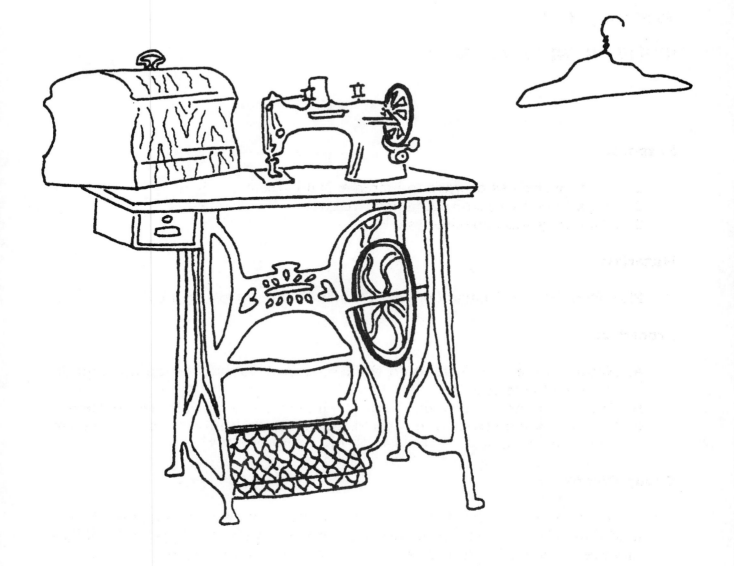

Something special someone made for me: _____

_____

Something I made for someone else: _____

_____

_____

Exercise 43

STEPS TO SELF-ESTEEM

Purpose:

1. Raise awareness of ways to increase self-esteem.
2. Instill hope by encouraging positive goals.
3. Promote group cohesiveness.

Materials:

Photocopy of the illustration for each member; pencils and crayons.

Procedure:

A. Materials are distributed and the leader or a member reads the caption about self-esteem.
B. The leader encourages members to tell about ways to raise self-esteem.
C. Members are instructed to write ideas for improving their own self-esteem on the stair steps.

Group Discussion:

It is important in this exercise that a range of realistic suggestions are made which will encourage members to build self-esteem. Suggestions might include participating in available activities, greeting someone pleasantly at mealtime, or paying special attention to grooming. Each member is asked to choose one idea to try in the next week.

The leader encourages reminiscence by asking members if they have lived in homes with stairways. Members are invited to share memories about stairs, banisters, and under-the-stair closets. Reminiscing about a common subject helps to build trust and group cohesiveness.

Steps to Self-Esteem

Good self-esteem is important in maintaining healthy attitudes and positive ways of coping with life's challenges. When self-esteem is low, it is more difficult to face the problems of daily living. People never outgrow their need to work on strengthening self-esteem.

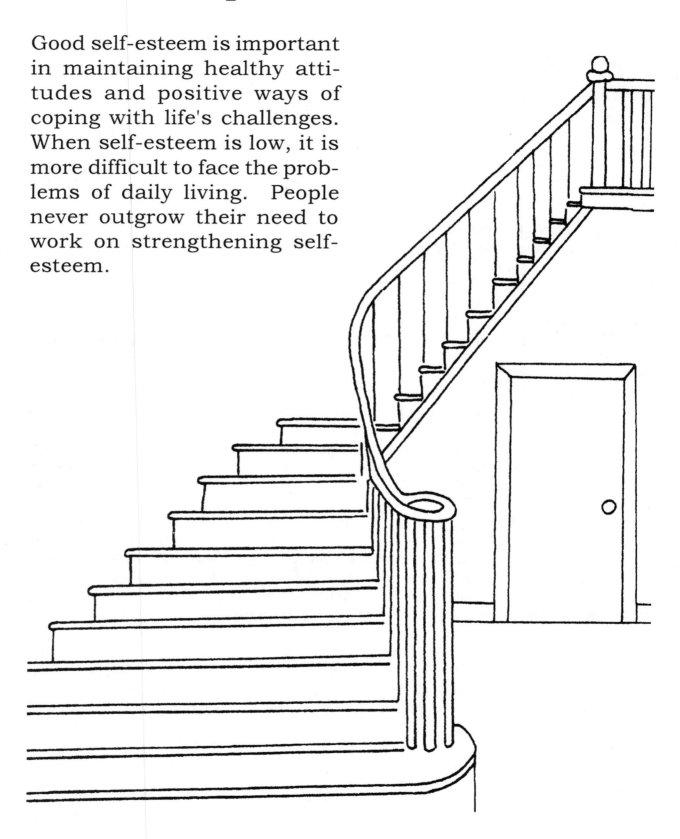

Exercise 44

GIVING THANKS

Purpose:

1. Emphasize positive thinking.
2. Strengthen identity and self-concept by sharing personal preferences.

Materials:

Old magazines, scissors, glue, felt pens, pencils, and posterboard (orange is effective for a Thanksgiving poster; however, this exercise can be used any time of the year).

Procedure:

A. Members are asked to cut pictures out of magazines to illustrate something they are thankful for. (If members are unable to use scissors, pre-cut pictures may be provided, or members who can use scissors can be asked to help those members who have difficulty.)
B. Label the poster: "We are thankful for. . . ." Glue the pictures chosen by members on the posterboard. Members are asked to sign their names on the poster beside pictures they have selected. (If a picture cannot be found to represent something a member is thankful for, the idea can be written with felt pen between the pictures.)

Group Discussion:

It is important to broaden the scope of thankfulness as much as possible. Small everyday events and pleasures should not be overlooked, such as coffee in the morning, shelter, a firm mattress, and beautiful sunsets. This exercise may be helpful for members with a negative outlook or those who are suffering from depression. Adding members' names under the pictures they have selected enhances identity and feelings of inclusiveness.

Variations:

Each member is given a photocopy of "We are thankful for. . . ." and asked to complete the list. Members may draw pictures in the margins to illustrate their ideas.

We are thankful for. . . .

_____

_____

_____

_____

_____

_____

_____

_____

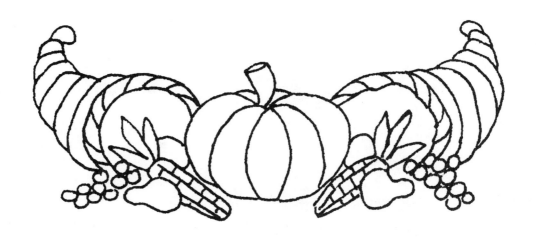

Exercise 45

WELLSPRINGS OF KNOWLEDGE

Purpose:

1. Encourage motivation by increasing knowledge of available resources.
2. Share background information to promote feelings of belonging.

Materials:

One photocopy of the illustration for each member; pencils and crayons.

Procedure:

A. Materials are distributed and members are asked to share memories and associations to the picture of the well. Some members may recall pumping water, drawing water from a well, or carrying water in long buckets.
B. The sentence fragment on the illustration is read aloud. Members are asked to describe what they think "Wellsprings of Knowledge" might refer to. Examples might include knowledgeable people, schools, or libraries.
C. The leader encourages members to think about "Wellsprings of Knowledge" in their own lives and to write their ideas in the blank.
D. Members may color the picture if they wish.

Group Discussion:

Members share their pictures and ideas about "Wellsprings of Knowledge" in their lives.

The leader points out that increasing one's knowledge is a lifetime process. Members are encouraged to tell about subjects they would like to learn more about. The leader and members brainstorm ideas on how to acquire information about the subjects named.

This exercise may enhance motivation and interest in the members' daily life. It is also useful in raising awareness of available resources for learning.

Wellsprings of Knowledge

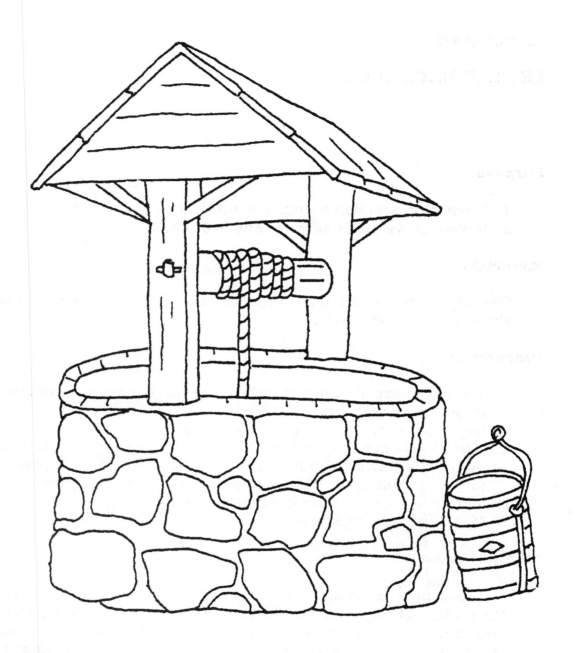

A wellspring of knowledge in my life was: _____

_____

_____

Exercise 46

LETTER EXCHANGE

Purpose:

1. Promote interaction to increase relatedness.
2. Increase awareness of the needs of others.

Materials:

One photocopy of the illustration for each member; pencils and crayons; slips of paper and a hat or box.

Procedure:

A. The leader explains that members are going to write letters to each other. Photocopies of the letter are distributed.
B. Members draw each other's names from a hat.
C. Using the photocopy, each member completes a letter to the member whose name was drawn. Members are asked to volunteer to help those who have difficulty writing so that each member completes a letter.
D. Members may color the illustration if they wish.
E. Members exchange letters.

Group Discussion:

Each member reads their letter and tells how they feel about the letter. The leader asks members to tell how they received mail in the past and whether they ever received a very important letter. Members are encouraged to share memories about the illustrations. Members are asked to describe the current procedure for sending and receiving mail.

This exercise is useful in promoting group cohesiveness. Withdrawn members often feel a greater sense of belonging after they give and receive a group letter.

Letter Exchange

Dear _____ ,

I'm glad to see you in the group because:

_____

_____

I like your: _____

_____

I hope your day is filled with: _____

_____

_____

Thank you for coming to the group and I hope to see you here again.

Warm regards,

_____

Exercise 47

WEATHERING HARD TIMES

Purpose:

1. Reveal personal history to increase feelings of belonging.
2. Share stories of survival to emphasize strengths and positive coping.

Materials:

One photocopy of the illustration for each member; fine-line colored felt pens or crayons.

Procedure:

A. While materials are being distributed, members are asked to think about storms, floods, hurricanes, or other stressful weather conditions they have experienced.
B. Members are asked to write their worst weather memory in the blank space.
C. Members may color the illustration or draw their own representation of a storm.

Group Discussion:

Members are asked to share memories about difficult weather they have encountered. Those who have colored or drawn show their pictures.

The leader asks each member to name coping skills used to survive fierce weather conditions.

Older adults often rely on coping skills they found useful earlier in life. Exploring these coping skills may help group members feel more effectual in solving current problems.

Weathering Hard Times

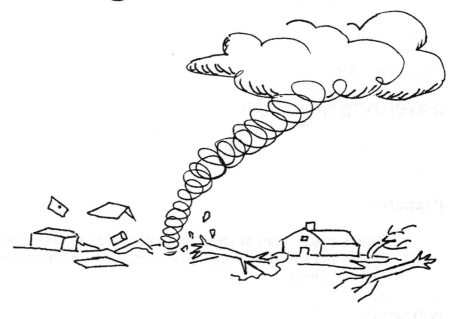

The worst weather condition I have experienced:

_____

_____

_____

_____

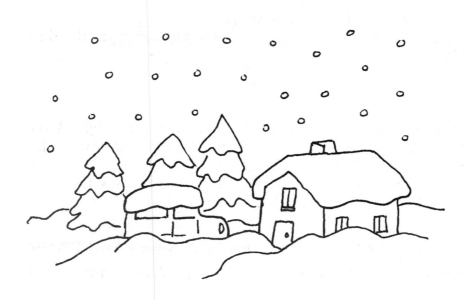

Exercise 48

FRIENDSHIP PIZZA

Purpose:

1. Raise awareness of the characteristics of friendly relationships.
2. Share personal history of important friendships to increase understanding of others.

Materials:

One photocopy of the illustration for each group member; crayons or colored felt pens, pencils, and scissors. ***Optional:*** posterboard and glue.

Procedure:

A. The leader explains that a good friendship is similar to a good pizza, in that certain ingredients are important.
B. Members are asked to tell what characteristics they think are important to a good friendship.
C. Materials are distributed and the leader tells members that they are going to make a "Friendship Pizza" to illustrate their ideas about friendship.
D. Members are asked to list characteristics of friendship that are important to them on the blanks in their pizza slice. Assistance is given to members who do not write.
E. Members may color the pizza slices if they wish.
F. The pizza slices are cut out and joined into a whole pizza during the discussion described below.

Group Discussion:

Members present their illustrations and ideas about friendship. After each presentation, the member's "pizza slice" is displayed in the center of the table, so that together, the slices form a whole pizza.

Members are asked to share about important friendships they have experienced, including current friendships.

The leader asks members for suggestions on how to encourage friendly attitudes in their present living situation.

Sharing about characteristics of friendship and friendships of the past may raise awareness of current opportunities for relating to others.

Variation:

The pizza slice illustrations can be glued onto posterboard with the title "Friendship Pizza."

Friendship Pizza

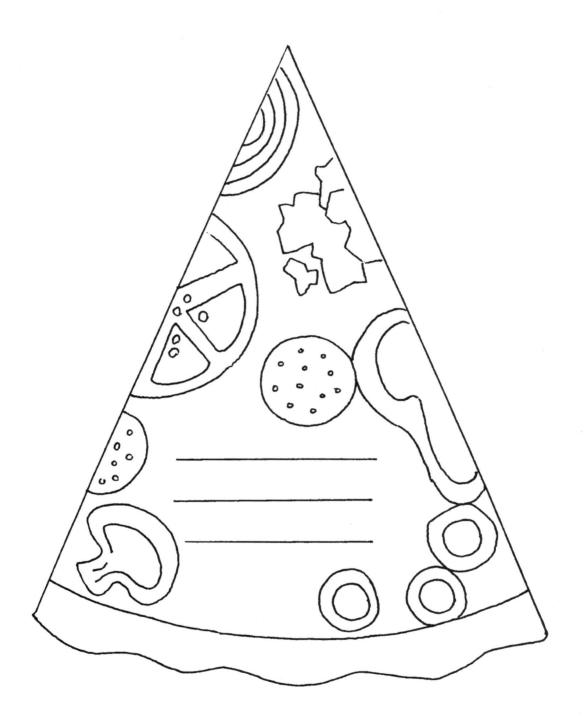

Exercise 49

DISTANT LOVED ONES

Purpose:

1. Encourage expressions of feelings about loved ones who live far away.
2. Promote positive coping with feelings of loss through supportive sharing of feelings.

Materials:

One photocopy of the illustration for each group member; crayons or fine-line colored felt pens. ***Optional:*** red or pink posterboard, scissors, and glue.

Procedure:

A. Materials are distributed and the caption is read aloud.
B. Members are asked to tell what the saying could mean.
C. The leader encourages members to think about loved ones they miss.
D. Members are instructed to color the designs and write names of loved ones in the blank heart. Some members may wish to make their own designs on the blank heart.

Group Discussion:

Members display their hearts and tell about loved ones they miss. Sharing feelings helps to ease the burden of loneliness.

Variations:

If desired, the hearts can be cut out and glued onto colored posterboard with a copy of the caption as a title for the poster. If the hearts are to be glued onto a poster, it is more dramatic to leave the hearts white and color the designs or names on the hearts with fine-line colored felt pens. The photocopies can also be folded in half and used as cards.

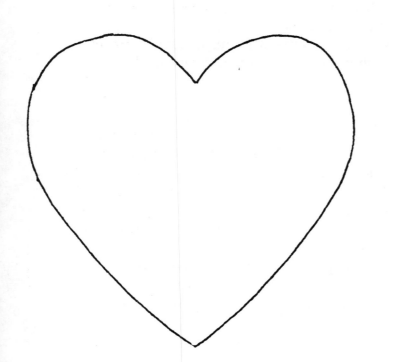 

Love
shortens the distance
between two hearts.

Exercise 50

SCHOOL DAYS

Purpose:

1. Share personal background to increase understanding of self and others.
2. Stimulate reminiscence to enhance feelings of identity and self-worth.

Materials:

One photocopy of the illustration for each group member; pencils and crayons.

Procedure:

A. While materials are passed out, members are asked to think about their school experiences.
B. The sentence fragments are read aloud and members are asked to describe the attitudes of the students in the picture.
C. Members are instructed to draw themselves in the empty desk and complete the sentences. Members may color the picture if they wish.

Group Discussion:

Members present their illustrations and sentences. The leader encourages members to share feelings and anecdotes about their school experiences. Members may discover they have feelings or experiences in common which help to build feelings of community. Members are asked if they would approach learning differently if they had it to do over. Current opportunities for learning can be discussed including current events, television, and radio.

School Days

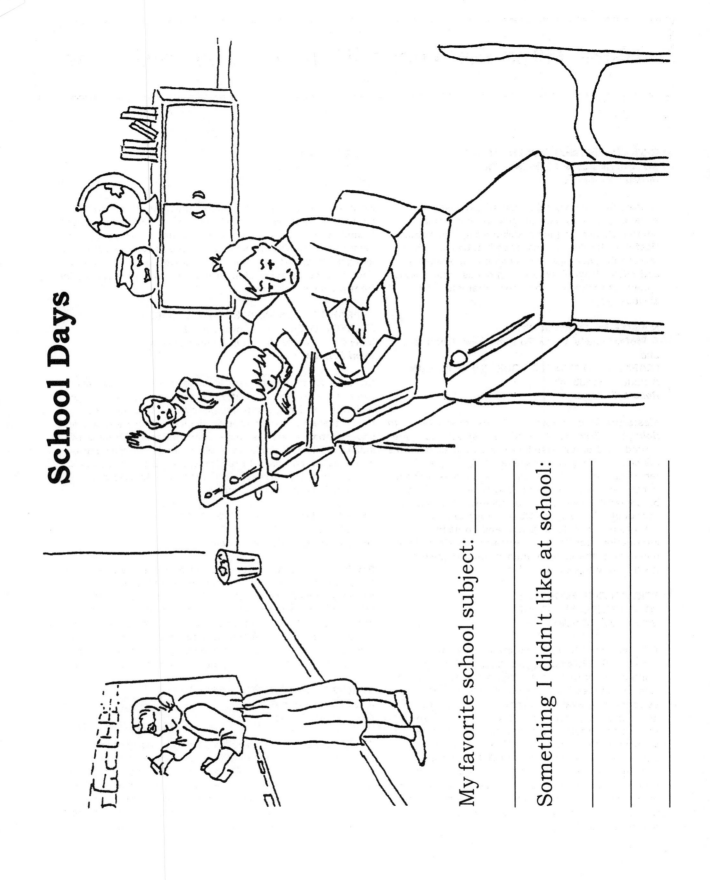

My favorite school subject: _____

Something I didn't like at school: _____

More Titles For Those Who Work With Groups

**GROUP EXERCISES FOR ENHANCING
SOCIAL SKILLS & SELF-ESTEEM**
SiriNam S. Khalsa

A uniquely creative collection of exercises for enhancing self-esteem utilizing proven social, emotional, and cognitive skill-building techniques. Useful in therapeutic, psychoeducational, and recreational settings with children, adolescents, and adults from diverse backgrounds with a wide variety of problems, concerns, interests, and abilities.

MASTERING CHRONIC PAIN:
A Professional's Guide To Behavioral Treatment
and
LEARNING TO MASTER YOUR CHRONIC PAIN:
A Patient Handbook
Robert N. Jamison

Mastering Chronic Pain: A Professional's Guide to Behavioral Treatment describes a structured, time-limited, and group-based pain program built on the principles of cognitive/behavioral therapy and rehabilitation. Includes many forms, illustrations, questionnaires, checklists, and letters which may be copied for use with your clients. The patient handbook, *Learning to Master Your Chronic Pain*, is written in simple language and contains information, forms, and exercises to help patients understand the phenomenon of chronic pain and learn new ways to control it.

**STRUCTURED ADOLESCENT
PSYCHOTHERAPY GROUPS**
Billie Farmer Corder

A "must read" book if you are a therapist who works with adolescents and their families. Contains how-to-do-it guidelines for each step in forming and leading a group including client selection and evaluation, goal setting, evaluating group process, relationships with a co-therapist, and much more. Offers concrete suggestions for working with "hard to reach" and difficult adolescents, providing feedback to parents, and dealing with administrative, legal, and ethical issues. Includes immediately usable examples of many forms, contracts, letters, rating scales, co-therapist rating forms, records, handouts, and group exercises.

CREATIVE THERAPY
Volumes I, II, & III
Jane Dossick & Eugene Shea

Each volume in this unique series presents 52 different, innovative, field-tested, and ready-to-use group exercises. Complete directions for the group leader are included with each exercise. These techniques have proved effective for all ages, from children over six to adolescents to adults. Each volume contains all new exercises with no duplication from previous volumes.

**THERAPEUTIC EXERCISES FOR VICTIMIZED &
NEGLECTED GIRLS:** Applications for
Individual, Family, & Group Psychotherapy
Pearl Berman

Contains 27 structured and focused therapeutic exercises designed to improve the effectiveness of your work with victimized and neglected girls in individual, group, and family therapy. Offers specific guidelines for selecting and implementing exercises focused on the specific needs of individual clients. **Includes a client handbook that can be photocopied** and used to reinforce the concepts and skills covered in the exercises. Skill-building exercises are presented, with full instructions.

**ASSESSMENT AND TREATMENT OF
ADOLESCENT SEX OFFENDERS**
Garry P. Perry & Janet Orchard

Provides invaluable guidance on effective assessment and treatment of adolescent sex offenders and their families. Provides procedures for classifying offenders, specific offender interview strategies, parent interview guidelines, and a checklist of risk factors. A group therapy approach is presented along with techniques for maximizing the long-term effects of various interventions. This book's practical advice will also be useful in your work with adult offenders.

STRESS MANAGEMENT TRAINING:
A Group Leader's Guide
Nancy Norvell & Dale Belles

This practical guide will help you define the concept of stress for group members and teach them various intervention techniques ranging from relaxation training to communication skills. Includes specific exercises, visual aids, stress response index, stress analysis form, and surveys for evaluating program effectiveness. Clinicians can easily modify these techniques for use with individual clients.

To receive more information, please complete and return the form on the back of this page ⟶

IF YOU FOUND THIS BOOK USEFUL...

...ight want to know more about our other titles.

...or a complete listing of our publications, please send us the following information. You may fold this sheet to make a postpa... reply envelope. If you ordered this book from Professional Resource Press, your name is already on our preferred custom... mailing list and you do not need to return this form to receive future catalogs.

Name _____
PLEASE PRINT

Address _____

Address _____

City/St/Zip _____

This address is my ☐home ☐office

I am a: ___Psychologist; ___Marriage & Family Therapist; ___School Psychologist; ___Clinical Social Worker; ___Mental Health Counselor; ___Psychiatrist; ___Other (please describe)_____

GWW...

Please fold on this line and the solid line below, tape (DO NOT STAPLE), and mail.

Please fold on this line and the solid line above, tape (DO NOT STAPLE), and mail.

NO POSTAGE NECESSARY IF MAILED IN THE UNITED STATES

BUSINESS REPLY MAIL
FIRST CLASS MAIL   PERMIT NO 445   SARASOTA FL

POSTAGE WILL BE PAID BY ADDRESSEE

PROFESSIONAL RESOURCE PRESS
PO BOX 15560
SARASOTA FL 34277-9900

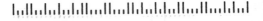